How to Survive a Nuclear War

Crafted by Skriuwer

Table of Contents

6. Surviving the First Week

6.1 Maintaining Your Shelter: Daily Routines and Checks

6.2 Resource Management: Rationing Food and Water

6.3 Staying Informed: Gathering News and Updates

6.4 Hygiene and Sanitation in a Confined Space

6.5 Planning for the Long-Term: What Comes Next?

7. Long-Term Survival Strategies

7.1 Finding Safe Water Sources

7.2 Growing and Sourcing Food Post-Attack

7.3 Establishing a New Normal: Daily Life After a Nuclear War

7.4 Staying Healthy: Preventing Disease and Injury

7.5 Rebuilding and Reconnecting with Society

8. Radiation: Understanding and Coping

8.1 What is Radiation? Types and Effects

8.2 Radiation Sickness: Symptoms and Treatments

8.3 Long-Term Health Risks: Cancer and Other Diseases

8.4 Reducing Radiation Exposure: Dos and Don'ts

8.5 Decontaminating Your Environment

9. Water and Food Safety in a Nuclear Environment

9.1 Identifying Contaminated Water Sources

9.2 Purifying Water: Techniques and Tools

9.3 Safe Food Sources: What to Eat and What to Avoid

9.4 Growing Food Post-Nuclear Attack

9.5 Storing and Preserving Food Safely

10. Communication and Information Gathering

10.1 Setting Up a Communication Network

10.2 Using Radios and Other Tools

10.3 Establishing Contact with Authorities

10.4 Finding Reliable Information: Avoiding Misinformation

10.5 The Role of Community Networks

16. The Role of Faith and Spirituality

16.1 Faith as a Source of Strength and Resilience

16.2 Spiritual Practices for Coping with Trauma

16.3 The Role of Religious Communities in Recovery

16.4 Ethical Dilemmas and Moral Decisions

16.5 Maintaining Hope and Finding Purpose

17. Government and Authority in Post-Nuclear Society

17.1 The Role of Government in Crisis Management

17.2 Martial Law and Civil Liberties: What to Expect

17.3 The Importance of Law and Order in Survival

17.4 The Role of International Organizations

17.5 Preparing for Potential Government Failures

18. Ethics and Morality in Survival Situations

18.1 The Ethics of Survival: Difficult Decisions

18.2 Balancing Self-Preservation and Community Needs

18.3 The Role of Compassion and Humanity

18.4 Legal and Ethical Challenges in Post-Nuclear Society

18.5 Preparing for Ethical Challenges: Moral Readiness

19. Learning from History: Case Studies of Survival

19.1 Hiroshima and Nagasaki: Lessons from Survivors

19.2 The Cuban Missile Crisis: Avoiding Nuclear Catastrophe

19.3 Chernobyl and Fukushima: Lessons from Nuclear Disasters

19.4 The Cold War Bunkers: Preparedness and Paranoia

19.5 Modern Nuclear Threats: North Korea and Iran

20. Conclusion: Moving Forward in a Post-Nuclear World

20.1 Reflecting on the Lessons Learned

20.2 The Importance of Preparedness and Vigilance

20.3 Rebuilding a Better World: Hope and Optimism

20.4 The Future of Nuclear Weapons: Challenges and Opportunities

20.5 Final Thoughts: Surviving and Thriving

Chapter 1

Understanding the Threat of Nuclear War

The History of Nuclear Weapons

The history of nuclear weapons is a complex narrative that spans over a century, characterized by scientific breakthroughs, political tensions, and ethical dilemmas. The genesis of nuclear weapons can be traced back to the early 20th century when scientists began to unlock the secrets of atomic structure. In 1896, Henri Becquerel discovered radioactivity, a phenomenon that would later play a crucial role in nuclear fission. This discovery set the stage for further exploration by pioneers like Marie Curie and Ernest Rutherford, who deepened our understanding of atomic particles.

The breakthrough that would lead to the development of nuclear weapons came when physicists discovered nuclear fission. In 1938, German scientists Otto Hahn and Fritz Strassmann conducted experiments that revealed that when uranium atoms were bombarded with neutrons, they split into smaller atoms, releasing a massive amount of energy. This monumental finding was further elucidated by physicists Lise Meitner and Otto Frisch, who explained the process and its potential for a chain reaction. The implications were staggering: a small amount of fissile material could produce an explosion of unprecedented scale.

The outbreak of World War II catalyzed the race for nuclear weapon development. In the United States, fearing that Nazi Germany would develop an atomic bomb first, President Franklin D. Roosevelt initiated the Manhattan Project in 1942. This top-secret research and development project brought together some of the greatest scientific minds of the time, including J. Robert Oppenheimer, Enrico Fermi, and Richard Feynman. The project culminated in the successful detonation of the first atomic bomb, known as the Trinity Test, on July 16, 1945, in the New Mexico desert.

Just weeks later, in August 1945, the United States dropped two atomic bombs on Japan—Hiroshima on August 6 and Nagasaki on August 9. These bombings resulted in the immediate deaths of approximately 200,000 people, with countless others suffering from radiation sickness and long-term health effects. The bombings effectively brought an end to World War II, but they also ushered in a new era marked by the specter of nuclear warfare.

The post-war landscape was dominated by the Cold War, a period characterized by intense rivalry between the United States and the Soviet Union. Both nations engaged in an arms race to develop more powerful nuclear arsenals, leading to the creation of hydrogen bombs—thermonuclear weapons that are significantly more destructive than atomic bombs. This arms race prompted the development of doctrines such as Mutually Assured Destruction (MAD), which posited that the full-scale use of nuclear weapons by two or more opposing sides would result in the total annihilation of both the attacker and the defender, thereby deterring direct conflict.

The proliferation of nuclear weapons was not limited to the superpowers; other nations, including the United Kingdom, France, China, India, Pakistan, and more recently, North Korea and Iran, have developed nuclear capabilities. Each new nuclear state has added layers of complexity to international relations, often leading to tense standoffs and crises.

In response to the growing nuclear threat, several international treaties were established, such as the Nuclear Non-Proliferation Treaty (NPT) of 1968, aimed at preventing the spread of nuclear weapons and promoting peaceful uses of nuclear energy. Despite these efforts, the risk of nuclear conflict remains a persistent global concern, exacerbated by geopolitical tensions, regional conflicts, and the potential for rogue states or non-state actors to acquire nuclear technology.

In conclusion, the history of nuclear weapons is a multifaceted tale of scientific ingenuity, military strategy, and ethical considerations. As we navigate the complexities of the modern world, understanding this history is crucial for assessing the ongoing risks and responsibilities associated with nuclear capabilities. The legacy of nuclear weapons continues to influence global politics, security, and the collective moral conscience of humanity.

The Current Global Nuclear Arsenal

The existence of nuclear weapons remains one of the most pressing challenges in global security. As of October 2023, nine countries possess nuclear arsenals, each with varying capabilities, policies, and doctrines regarding the use of these weapons. Understanding the current global nuclear arsenal is crucial for assessing the geopolitical landscape and the potential for nuclear conflict.

1. Countries with Nuclear Capabilities

The nine nuclear-armed states include the United States, Russia, China, France, the United Kingdom, India, Pakistan, Israel, and North Korea. Each of these nations has developed its nuclear weapons program under different historical, political, and strategic motives.

- **United States:** The U.S. was the first country to develop nuclear weapons, successfully testing its first bomb in 1945. Today, it maintains a significant arsenal, with approximately 3,750 nuclear warheads. The U.S. nuclear policy is built around deterrence and includes a triad of delivery systems: land-based intercontinental ballistic missiles (ICBMs), submarine-launched ballistic missiles (SLBMs), and strategic bombers.

- **Russia:** Following the U.S., Russia (formerly the Soviet Union) developed its nuclear capabilities, which are now estimated at around 6,375 warheads. Russia's nuclear strategy emphasizes the need for a robust second-strike capability, ensuring that any adversary knows a nuclear response is inevitable in the event of an attack.

- **China:** China has been expanding its nuclear arsenal, which is estimated to comprise around 410 warheads. China's nuclear posture has historically been characterized by a no-first-use policy, indicating a commitment not to use nuclear weapons unless first attacked by an adversary.

- **France and the United Kingdom:** Both countries possess nuclear arsenals of around 290 and 225 warheads, respectively. France's nuclear strategy is integrated into its overall defense policy, while the UK's arsenal is primarily seen as a deterrent against major threats to national security.

- **India and Pakistan:** Both nations developed nuclear weapons amid regional tensions. India has approximately 160 warheads, while Pakistan possesses about 170. Their nuclear doctrines are aimed at deterring each other, with India focusing on a no-first-use policy and Pakistan maintaining a more ambiguous stance.

- **Israel:** While Israel has never officially confirmed its nuclear arsenal, estimates suggest it has around 90 warheads. Israel's nuclear policy is rooted in ambiguity, which serves as a deterrent against existential threats in a hostile regional environment.

- **North Korea:** North Korea's nuclear program has rapidly advanced, especially under the leadership of Kim Jong-un. The country is believed to possess around 50 to 75 warheads and continues to develop its delivery systems, including intercontinental ballistic missiles capable of reaching the U.S. mainland.

2. Global Trends and Implications

The proliferation of nuclear weapons raises critical concerns regarding global security. The ongoing modernization of nuclear arsenals, particularly by the United States and Russia, has led to an arms race reminiscent of the Cold War era. Furthermore, the potential for nuclear proliferation in volatile regions, such as the Middle East, poses risks of nuclear escalation and conflict.

Moreover, the strategic doctrines of these nuclear-armed states vary significantly, influencing their policies on deterrence and potential use of nuclear weapons. The lack of comprehensive disarmament agreements and the stagnation of international arms control efforts leave the global community vulnerable to the risks associated with nuclear weapons.

In summary, the current global nuclear arsenal reflects a complex interplay of historical legacies, national security strategies, and geopolitical dynamics. Understanding these factors is essential for mitigating the risks associated with nuclear weapons and fostering a safer, more secure world. As the landscape evolves, ongoing dialogue and diplomatic efforts are critical to reducing the likelihood of nuclear conflict and advancing global disarmament initiatives.

The Political Landscape: Tensions and Alliances

The political landscape surrounding nuclear weapons is a complex interplay of international relations, historical grievances, and strategic interests that significantly influence the likelihood of nuclear conflict. Nuclear weapons are not merely military tools; they are powerful symbols of national strength and deterrence, deeply embedded in the fabric of global politics. Understanding this landscape requires examining the tensions and alliances that shape nuclear discourse and policy.

Historical Context

The development of nuclear weapons during World War II marked a pivotal moment in global politics, ushering in the Cold War era characterized by ideological rivalry between the United States and the Soviet Union. This rivalry entrenched a system of deterrence based on mutually assured destruction (MAD), where both nations possessed enough nuclear capability to obliterate each other in the event of a conflict. The legacy of this historical context continues to echo in contemporary geopolitical tensions, particularly among nuclear-armed states.

Current Tensions

Modern geopolitical tensions are often rooted in historical conflicts, territorial disputes, and ideological divides. For instance, the ongoing tensions between North Korea and the United States highlight how nuclear ambitions can exacerbate international crises. North Korea's pursuit of nuclear capabilities is driven by a desire for regime security and international recognition, leading to a cycle of provocations and military posturing. Similarly, the tensions between India and Pakistan, both nuclear-armed states, are fueled by historical animosities and territorial disputes, particularly over Kashmir. These situations underscore the precariousness of nuclear peace, where misunderstandings or miscalculations can quickly escalate into conflict.

Alliances and Strategic Partnerships
Nuclear alliances play a crucial role in shaping the political landscape. The North Atlantic Treaty Organization (NATO), for example, serves as a collective defense arrangement that enhances the deterrence posture of member states against potential nuclear threats from adversaries, such as Russia. The U.S. extends its nuclear umbrella to allied nations, reinforcing the strategic calculus of deterrence in Europe and Asia. Similarly, the U.S.-Japan and U.S.-South Korea alliances are pivotal in countering North Korean threats, emphasizing the importance of international partnerships in nuclear strategy.

Conversely, the rise of new alliances among non-Western countries, such as the Sino-Russian partnership, presents a counterbalance to U.S. influence and complicates the nuclear landscape. This alliance has led to increased military cooperation and joint exercises, signaling a unified stance against perceived Western aggression. The dynamics of these alliances, therefore, can either stabilize or destabilize the nuclear order, depending on how they interact with existing rivalries and conflicts.

The Role of International Organizations
International organizations, particularly the United Nations (UN) and the International Atomic Energy Agency (IAEA), play critical roles in mitigating nuclear tensions through diplomacy and arms control initiatives. Treaties such as the Treaty on the Non-Proliferation of Nuclear Weapons (NPT) aim to prevent the spread of nuclear weapons and promote disarmament. However, the effectiveness of these treaties often hinges on the political will of nuclear-armed states to comply with their obligations. The erosion of trust among nations, as seen in the breakdown of the Intermediate-Range Nuclear Forces Treaty (INF), highlights the fragility of diplomatic efforts in a tense political climate.

Conclusion
Ultimately, the political landscape surrounding nuclear weapons is a dynamic and multifaceted environment influenced by historical grievances, strategic alliances, and the ever-present threat of conflict. As nations navigate their interests and security concerns, the likelihood of nuclear conflict remains contingent upon the ability of global actors to foster dialogue, build trust, and engage in cooperative security arrangements. Understanding these complexities is essential for

developing strategies that seek to reduce tensions and promote a more stable nuclear order in an increasingly interconnected world.

The Science of Nuclear Explosions

Nuclear weapons are among the most powerful and devastating tools of warfare ever created, harnessing the energy released from nuclear reactions to produce explosive force. To understand nuclear explosions, it is essential to delve into the underlying science, which primarily revolves around two processes: nuclear fission and nuclear fusion.

Nuclear Fission is the process by which the nucleus of an atom splits into smaller parts, releasing a tremendous amount of energy. This reaction is the principle behind atomic bombs, such as those dropped on Hiroshima and Nagasaki. The most commonly used fissile materials in these bombs are isotopes of uranium (U-235) and plutonium (Pu-239). When a neutron collides with the nucleus of a fissile atom, it can cause the nucleus to become unstable and split, releasing additional neutrons and a significant amount of energy in the form of a shockwave and heat. This release of neutrons can then initiate a chain reaction, where each fission event causes further fission in surrounding nuclei, leading to an exponential increase in energy release.

Nuclear Fusion, on the other hand, involves the combination of light atomic nuclei to form a heavier nucleus, a process that releases even more energy than fission. Fusion is the principle that powers the sun and other stars. In thermonuclear weapons, or hydrogen bombs, fusion reactions are triggered by the energy from an initial fission explosion. Isotopes of hydrogen, such as deuterium and tritium, are commonly used in fusion reactions. The heat and pressure generated by the fission explosion provide the necessary conditions for fusion to occur, resulting in an immensely powerful explosion.

The effects of a nuclear explosion can be categorized into immediate and secondary impacts, each with significant implications for human life and the environment.

1. Blast Wave: The explosive force from a nuclear detonation creates a blast wave that travels outward at high speed. This wave can demolish buildings, uproot trees, and cause extensive physical destruction over a wide area. The radius of destruction depends on the yield of the weapon, with larger bombs causing damage over several miles.

2. Thermal Radiation: A nuclear explosion generates an intense amount of heat, leading to thermal radiation that can cause severe burns and ignite fires at considerable distances from the blast site. The heat can cause third-degree burns to individuals many kilometers away, creating firestorms that can devastate urban areas.

3. Nuclear Fallout: Following the explosion, radioactive particles are released into the atmosphere and can descend back to the ground, a phenomenon known as fallout. This fallout can contaminate air, water, and soil, posing severe health risks, including acute radiation sickness and long-term effects such as cancer.

4. Electromagnetic Pulse (EMP): A nuclear explosion can also produce an EMP, a burst of electromagnetic radiation that can disrupt or destroy electronic devices and electrical infrastructure over a vast area. This effect can cripple communication systems and essential services, exacerbating the aftermath of the explosion.

5. Psychological Impact: The catastrophic nature of a nuclear explosion instills profound psychological fear and trauma. The immediate shock of the event, combined with the uncertainty of survival and the breakdown of societal structures, can lead to long-lasting mental health issues among survivors.

In conclusion, understanding the science behind nuclear explosions is critical for grasping their potential consequences. The combination of fission and fusion reactions, along with the immediate destructive effects and long-term implications of radiation exposure, highlights the need for preparedness and awareness in the face of the nuclear threat. As global tensions persist, educating oneself on the mechanics and effects of nuclear weapons remains an essential aspect of survival planning.

Assessing the Likelihood of Nuclear Conflict

In the contemporary geopolitical landscape, the specter of nuclear conflict looms ominously, driven by a complex interplay of international relations, national security policies, and regional tensions. This section aims to evaluate the current risks associated with nuclear conflict and the scenarios that could potentially trigger such an event, providing a deeper understanding of the factors at play.

Current Geopolitical Landscape

The geopolitical arena is marked by a resurgence of great power competition, particularly among the United States, Russia, and China. Each of these nations possesses substantial nuclear arsenals and has demonstrated a willingness to assert their national interests through military posturing. The deteriorating relationships between these powers have resulted in an arms race reminiscent of the Cold War era, with advancements in nuclear capabilities and military technologies escalating tensions.

Regional conflicts also contribute to the likelihood of nuclear conflict. For instance, the ongoing tensions in the Korean Peninsula, where North Korea has developed nuclear weapons and ballistic missile capabilities, pose a significant threat not only to regional stability but also to global security. The potential for miscalculation or miscommunication in a crisis situation raises the stakes, as any military confrontation could spiral into a nuclear exchange.

The Role of Alliances and Treaties

Nuclear alliances, such as NATO, play a critical role in the current landscape. The principle of nuclear deterrence relies on the assurance that an attack on one ally will invoke a response from others, potentially escalating to nuclear retaliation. However, this intricate web of alliances can also lead to misunderstandings and unintended escalations. The withdrawal of key players from disarmament treaties, such as the Intermediate-Range Nuclear Forces Treaty (INF), further complicates the dynamics, as it erodes trust and increases the potential for arms development.

The effectiveness of arms control agreements has diminished in recent years, with both the United States and Russia engaging in behaviors that undermine previous commitments. The New START treaty, which limits the number of deployed strategic nuclear warheads, faces uncertainties regarding its future, especially as relations between these powers continue to fray.

Technological Advancements and Cyber Threats

Technological advancements in missile defense systems, artificial intelligence, and cyber capabilities pose additional risks. The development of hypersonic weapons, designed to evade traditional missile defense systems, challenges existing deterrence strategies and could prompt preemptive strikes in a crisis. Furthermore, the vulnerability of nuclear command and control systems to cyberattacks raises the specter of unauthorized launches or accidental conflicts, amplifying the potential for miscalculation.

Assessing Risk Scenarios

Several scenarios could precipitate nuclear conflict, including:

1. Escalation of Regional Conflicts: A conventional military confrontation, such as a conflict in the South China Sea or between India and Pakistan, could escalate quickly, particularly if nuclear-armed states perceive their survival is at stake.

2. Accidental Launch: Technical malfunctions or human errors could inadvertently lead to a nuclear launch. The historical precedent of near-misses during the Cold War highlights the critical need for robust safeguards.

3. Terrorism and Non-State Actors: The potential for non-state actors to acquire nuclear materials or technology poses a significant threat. A terrorist group's ability to detonate a nuclear device could evoke immediate retaliatory measures from nuclear states.

4. Political Instability: Internal political turmoil within a nuclear-armed state could lead to the loss of control over nuclear arsenals, increasing the risk of use or proliferation.

5. Strategic Miscalculations: In high-stakes situations, leaders may misinterpret intentions or capabilities of adversaries, leading to decisions that could trigger nuclear conflict.

In conclusion, assessing the likelihood of nuclear conflict requires a thorough understanding of the current global dynamics, technological advancements, and the underlying political tensions. As nations navigate a precarious balance between deterrence and diplomacy, the need for robust communication, crisis management strategies, and renewed commitments to arms control has never been more urgent. The stakes are high, and the path forward necessitates vigilance, collaboration, and a commitment to preventing the unthinkable.

Chapter 2

Immediate Effects of a Nuclear Explosion

The Blast Wave

In the immediate aftermath of a nuclear explosion, one of the most devastating effects is the blast wave, a powerful shockwave generated by the rapid release of energy from the detonation. Understanding the characteristics of this blast wave is crucial for assessing the destruction radius and the immediate danger it poses to life and infrastructure.

Characteristics of the Blast Wave

The explosion of a nuclear weapon creates a fireball that expands outward at supersonic speeds, compressing the surrounding air and generating a shockwave. This blast wave propagates in all directions, with its intensity and impact diminishing as it travels further from the epicenter. The blast wave is characterized by a rapid increase in pressure followed by a swift drop, creating a powerful force that can obliterate buildings, shatter windows, and cause severe injuries or fatalities.

Destruction Radius

The destruction radius of a nuclear explosion varies significantly depending on the weapon's yield, measured in kilotons or megatons of TNT equivalent. For example, a 1-kiloton nuclear explosion produces a blast wave capable of causing significant destruction within a radius of approximately 1,000 feet (around 300 meters). In contrast, a 10-megaton explosion can devastate an area several miles in diameter.

The area of complete destruction, often referred to as the "ground zero," is where buildings are flattened, and survival is highly unlikely. Within this zone, the blast pressure can exceed 20 pounds per square inch (psi), sufficient to cause catastrophic damage to reinforced structures.

Immediate Effects of the Blast Wave

1. Structural Damage: Buildings, especially those not designed to withstand blasts, are susceptible to collapse. The majority of conventional structures within the primary destruction radius may be reduced to rubble, while more fortified buildings may suffer extensive damage but remain standing.

2. Injuries and Fatalities: The blast wave can cause a wide array of injuries, from blunt force trauma to lacerations from flying debris. Individuals in close proximity to the explosion may experience instantaneous death or severe injuries due to the pressure differential and the resulting impact.

3. Secondary Effects: The initial blast can trigger fires in surrounding areas, compounded by the thermal radiation emitted by the explosion. As buildings collapse, gas lines may rupture, leading to explosions and further fires, creating a chaotic and dangerous environment.

4. Psychological Impact: The shockwave produces not only physical destruction but also an overwhelming psychological impact on survivors. The noise generated by the explosion can exceed 200 decibels, contributing to auditory trauma and confusion. The fear and uncertainty following such an event can lead to panic, disorientation, and long-lasting psychological effects.

Conclusion
The blast wave from a nuclear explosion is a devastating force, characterized by its capacity to inflict immediate destruction and chaos within a significant radius. Understanding the dynamics of the blast wave—its formation, effects, and the potential for widespread devastation—is vital for preparing for and responding to a nuclear event. Preparedness efforts should include educating communities about the risks associated with nuclear detonations, creating emergency response plans, and fostering resilience in the face of such unprecedented challenges. In the grim reality of a nuclear explosion, knowledge and awareness can be critical tools in mitigating the impact of the blast wave on human life and infrastructure.

Thermal Radiation: Burns and Fires
Thermal radiation is one of the most immediate and devastating effects of a nuclear explosion, capable of inflicting severe injuries and widespread destruction. When a nuclear weapon detonates, it releases an immense amount of energy in the form of heat and light, generating temperatures that can exceed tens of millions of degrees Fahrenheit at the epicenter. This intense heat propagates outward, causing burns, igniting fires, and creating a perilous environment for anyone within the blast radius.

Mechanisms of Thermal Radiation
The thermal radiation emitted from a nuclear explosion primarily consists of infrared radiation, visible light, and ultraviolet radiation. The initial flash of light is observed as a blinding brilliance, often accompanied by a fireball that expands rapidly. This fireball radiates heat in all directions, resulting in intense thermal effects that can cause serious injury even at significant distances

from the explosion site. The severity of thermal burns is contingent on several factors, including distance from the blast, duration of exposure, and the presence of flammable materials.

Types of Burns
Burns caused by thermal radiation can be categorized into four degrees based on severity:

1. First-Degree Burns: These are superficial burns affecting only the outer layer of skin. Symptoms include redness, minor swelling, and pain, similar to a sunburn. While first-degree burns can be painful, they typically heal without medical intervention.

2. Second-Degree Burns: These burns penetrate deeper, affecting both the epidermis and part of the dermis. They can cause blisters, severe pain, and swelling. Second-degree burns often require medical treatment, especially if they cover a large area.

3. Third-Degree Burns: These are severe, full-thickness burns that destroy both layers of skin and may damage underlying tissues. The area may appear white, charred, or leathery, and is typically painless due to nerve damage. Third-degree burns necessitate immediate medical attention and can lead to significant complications, including infections and scarring.

4. Fourth-Degree Burns: The most severe type, these burns extend through the skin to deeper tissues, potentially affecting muscles, tendons, and bones. Fourth-degree burns are life-threatening and require extensive medical intervention, often involving surgery and rehabilitation.

Fires and Secondary Hazards
In addition to direct thermal burns, the heat generated by a nuclear explosion can ignite flammable materials, leading to widespread fires. These fires can spread rapidly, fueled by debris and structures in urban environments. The firestorms that may result can create their own weather systems, exacerbating destruction and complicating rescue and recovery efforts.

The combination of burns and fires can lead to a catastrophic situation. Individuals who survive the initial blast may find themselves in life-threatening circumstances due to the ensuing fires, which can cause smoke inhalation, further burns, and injuries related to collapsing structures.

Protective Measures
To mitigate the dangers of thermal radiation, it is essential to understand and prepare for potential exposure. If a nuclear explosion is imminent, individuals should seek shelter in a robust, insulated building away from windows and external walls. The use of protective clothing

and coverings can help shield the skin from burns. Additionally, having a well-stocked emergency kit with medical supplies, including burn dressings and ointments, can be invaluable in the aftermath of a blast.

In conclusion, the thermal radiation resulting from a nuclear explosion poses significant threats through direct burns and secondary fire hazards. Understanding these dangers is crucial for effective preparation and response strategies, as survival may depend on swift actions taken immediately following a nuclear event. Awareness of the potential for thermal injuries and the implementation of protective measures can significantly increase the chances of enduring such a catastrophic situation.

Nuclear Fallout: Radioactive Contamination

Nuclear fallout refers to the residual radioactive material propelled into the upper atmosphere following a nuclear explosion, which then descends back to Earth. This phenomenon is a critical concern in the event of a nuclear detonation, as it poses immediate and long-term health risks to populations, ecosystems, and infrastructure. Understanding the nature of nuclear fallout, its spread, and the associated dangers is essential for effective preparedness and response.

How Fallout Spreads

The spread of nuclear fallout is influenced by several factors, including the yield of the nuclear explosion, the altitude at which the detonation occurs, and prevailing weather conditions. When a nuclear bomb detonates, it creates a massive fireball that vaporizes nearby materials, including soil, buildings, and vegetation. This vaporized material, along with radioactive isotopes produced during the fission process, is thrust into the atmosphere.

Once in the air, these particles can be carried by wind currents over vast distances, sometimes hundreds of miles from the blast site. Fallout can settle in various forms: as larger particles that fall close to the explosion site (known as "early fallout"), or as smaller, more dispersed particles that can travel further before descending (known as "delayed fallout"). The timing and location of rainfall can further impact fallout distribution, as precipitation can wash radioactive materials from the atmosphere, causing them to settle on the ground.

Immediate Dangers of Fallout

The immediate dangers posed by nuclear fallout primarily stem from its radioactive nature. Fallout consists of various isotopes with differing half-lives and biological impacts. Some of the most concerning isotopes include cesium-137, strontium-90, and iodine-131. Each of these isotopes can have severe health implications:

1. Radiation Exposure: Direct exposure to fallout can lead to acute radiation sickness, which manifests as nausea, vomiting, fatigue, and, in severe cases, death. The severity of symptoms depends on the dose of radiation received. High doses can cause immediate health effects, while lower doses may increase the risk of cancer over time.

2. Contamination of Food and Water: Fallout can contaminate the environment, affecting soil, water supplies, and food sources. Radioactive particles can settle on crops and livestock, rendering them unsafe for consumption. Water sources can also become contaminated, requiring emergency purification measures.

3. Long-Term Health Risks: The long-term health risks associated with fallout exposure include an increased likelihood of developing cancers, particularly thyroid cancer due to iodine-131 uptake by the thyroid gland. Other potential long-term effects include damage to the immune system and genetic mutations.

Protective Measures

In the wake of a nuclear explosion, immediate protective measures are vital to mitigate the effects of fallout. These include:

- **Sheltering in Place:** Staying indoors, especially in basements or windowless rooms, can significantly reduce exposure. Sealing windows and doors can help prevent fallout particles from entering.

- **Monitoring Radiation Levels:** Use of portable radiation detectors can help assess contamination levels and determine safe times for evacuation or outdoor activities.

- **Decontamination:** If exposed to fallout, it is crucial to decontaminate by removing clothing and washing thoroughly to minimize radiation exposure.

- **Emergency Supplies:** Stockpiling potassium iodide can help protect the thyroid from iodine-131 absorption. Additionally, having access to clean food and water is essential for survival.

In conclusion, understanding the dynamics of nuclear fallout and its immediate dangers is critical for effective disaster preparedness and response. By taking appropriate measures to shelter, monitor, and decontaminate, individuals and communities can significantly reduce their risk of radiation exposure and its associated health effects following a nuclear event.

The Electromagnetic Pulse (EMP): Disrupting Technology

An Electromagnetic Pulse (EMP) is a burst of electromagnetic radiation that can disrupt or damage electronic devices and electrical infrastructure. This phenomenon can occur naturally, such as during a solar flare, or artificially through a nuclear explosion detonated at high altitudes. Understanding the effects of an EMP is critical, particularly in the context of a nuclear war, as it poses a unique threat to modern technology and societal infrastructure.

Nature and Mechanism of EMP

When a nuclear weapon detonates at high altitude, it produces a powerful pulse of electromagnetic radiation that radiates outward, affecting a vast area. The pulse travels at the speed of light, generating electric and magnetic fields that induce electrical currents in conductive materials. This can overload and damage electronic circuits, leading to widespread failures of electrical systems.

An EMP can be categorized into three components: E1, E2, and E3. E1 is a fast pulse that can disrupt microelectronics and communication systems, while E2 is similar to lightning and can affect power grids. E3 is a slower pulse that can damage long-line electrical systems, such as power transmission lines. The combination of these effects can result in catastrophic disruptions to electrical grids and technological systems essential for modern life.

Impact on Electronics and Infrastructure

The potential impact of an EMP on electronics is profound. Devices such as computers, smartphones, radios, and even newer vehicles equipped with electronic controls could be rendered inoperative. The E1 component, which occurs within nanoseconds, is particularly damaging to microelectronics, causing permanent damage to components that are integral to communication and data processing.

Infrastructure, particularly power grids, is highly vulnerable to EMPs. The E2 and E3 components can induce currents in power lines, potentially causing transformers to fail. In the aftermath of an EMP event, the cascading failures of electrical systems could lead to widespread blackouts, affecting everything from healthcare facilities to water supply systems. The restoration of these systems could take weeks, if not months, depending on the scale of the damage and the availability of replacement parts.

Societal Consequences

The societal consequences of an EMP event are far-reaching. The immediate loss of communication capabilities would hinder emergency response efforts and disrupt daily life.

Essential services such as transportation, food distribution, and emergency healthcare could be severely affected, leading to panic and chaos among the population.

Moreover, the psychological impact of an EMP cannot be understated. The sudden loss of technology that individuals rely on for information, communication, and comfort can lead to heightened anxiety and fear. The disruption of social networks, as people are unable to contact loved ones or access news, can exacerbate feelings of isolation and uncertainty.

Preparing for EMP Threats

Preparation for an EMP event requires a multifaceted approach. Individuals and communities can take proactive steps, such as creating EMP-proof shelters for essential electronics, developing communication plans that rely on non-electronic methods, and stockpiling supplies that do not require electricity for preservation. Additionally, investing in Faraday cages—enclosures that protect electronic devices from electromagnetic interference—can be a practical measure for safeguarding crucial technology.

Governments must also consider the implications of EMP threats in their emergency preparedness plans. This includes investing in hardening critical infrastructure against EMP effects, conducting public awareness campaigns about the potential risks, and promoting community resilience through education and preparedness training.

Conclusion

In summary, the threat of an Electromagnetic Pulse, particularly in the context of a nuclear event, poses significant challenges to modern society. Understanding its mechanisms, potential impacts, and the necessary preparations can help mitigate the risks associated with this disruptive force. By fostering awareness and resilience, individuals and communities can better navigate the uncertainties of a post-EMP world.

Psychological Impact: Coping with Shock and Fear

The prospect of a nuclear attack is one of the most daunting scenarios one can contemplate. The psychological impact of such an event can be profound and long-lasting. Understanding how to mentally prepare for and respond to the shock and fear that accompany the threat of nuclear war is crucial for survival—both in the immediate aftermath and in the long term.

Understanding Shock and Fear

Shock is a natural initial response to trauma, characterized by feelings of disbelief, confusion, and emotional numbness. Fear, on the other hand, is a more sustained emotional state, often fueled by uncertainty about the future, the safety of loved ones, and the potential for widespread destruction. Recognizing these emotions as normal reactions to an extraordinary situation can help individuals process their feelings more effectively.

Mental Preparation Before an Attack

1. Education and Awareness: Knowledge about the risks, effects, and survival strategies concerning nuclear attacks can empower individuals. Understanding the science behind nuclear explosions, the likely immediate effects, and the steps to take can mitigate fear. Familiarizing oneself with resources—like emergency plans and survival guides—can foster a sense of control.

2. Mindfulness and Stress Reduction Techniques: Practicing mindfulness, meditation, and deep-breathing exercises can help maintain emotional balance in the face of anxiety. These techniques can be practiced daily to build resilience and improve coping mechanisms.

3. Developing a Support Network: Building relationships with family, friends, and community members can provide a safety net in times of crisis. Open dialogues about fears and concerns can foster stronger bonds and promote collective coping strategies.

4. Creating a Survival Plan: Having a well-thought-out survival plan can significantly reduce anxiety. This plan should include emergency contacts, communication strategies, and clearly defined roles within your family or group. Knowing you have a plan can alleviate feelings of helplessness.

Responding to an Attack
In the event of a nuclear attack, the immediate psychological response can be overwhelming. However, knowing how to cope can make a significant difference.

1. Recognize Your Emotions: Allow yourself to feel and express emotions. It's essential to acknowledge feelings of fear and shock without judgment. Writing in a journal or talking to someone can be therapeutic.

2. Follow the Survival Plan: In the chaos that follows an attack, sticking to the survival plan can provide a sense of purpose and direction. Focus on actionable steps—seeking shelter, securing supplies, and checking on loved ones.

3. Limit Exposure to News: While it is essential to stay informed, excessive exposure to distressing news can exacerbate anxiety. Set boundaries around media consumption, and rely on trusted sources for updates.

4. Practice Grounding Techniques: Grounding techniques can help manage panic and anxiety. Techniques include focusing on your breath, identifying objects in your immediate environment, or engaging in simple physical activities.

Long-Term Coping Strategies
The aftermath of a nuclear attack can leave lasting psychological scars. Long-term coping strategies are vital for recovery.

1. Seek Professional Help: Mental health professionals can provide essential support in processing trauma. Counseling or therapy can help individuals work through their feelings and develop coping strategies tailored to their needs.

2. Engage in Community Support: Rebuilding social ties and participating in community activities can promote healing. Sharing experiences with others who have faced similar challenges can foster a sense of belonging.

3. Establish Routines: Creating daily routines can instill a sense of normalcy in a chaotic environment. Focus on basic self-care, including nutrition, exercise, and rest, as these can greatly impact mental well-being.

4. Foster Resilience: Emphasize personal strengths and resilience. Reflecting on past challenges and how you overcame them can build confidence in your ability to cope with future adversities.

In sum, preparing mentally for a nuclear attack involves a combination of education, emotional awareness, and practical strategies. By understanding the psychological impact of such a crisis and implementing coping mechanisms, individuals can enhance their resilience and ability to navigate a post-nuclear world.

Chapter 3

Preparing for a Nuclear War

Building a Survival Plan: Assessing Risks and Needs

Creating a personalized survival strategy is a vital first step in preparing for a potential nuclear event. The process begins with a thorough assessment of risks and needs that are unique to your situation, environment, and community. This assessment allows you to develop a tailored plan that not only addresses immediate threats but also prepares you for long-term survival in a post-nuclear world.

Understanding Risks

The first component of your survival plan involves identifying the specific risks associated with nuclear conflict in your area. This may include proximity to military bases or nuclear facilities, the likelihood of political tensions escalating into conflict, and the geographical features that could affect fallout spread, such as wind patterns and elevation. Consider historical contexts as well; regions with a history of military conflict may be more prone to nuclear threats.

Additionally, evaluate other potential risks that could compound the effects of a nuclear event. These might include natural disasters (like earthquakes or floods), economic instability, or civil unrest. Each of these factors can significantly affect your survival strategy and resource allocation.

Assessing Personal Needs

Next, it's crucial to assess your personal needs and those of your household. Consider the number of individuals in your household, their ages, medical conditions, and any special requirements. For example, infants may need formula, while elderly family members might require medications or mobility aids. Compile a comprehensive list of supplies tailored to these needs, including food, water, medical supplies, and sanitation products.

Think about the psychological and emotional needs of your household as well. A nuclear event can create significant stress and trauma; therefore, developing coping strategies and maintaining open lines of communication will be essential for mental resilience.

Inventorying Resources

With a clear understanding of risks and needs, conduct an inventory of your current resources. This includes assessing your emergency supplies, food storage, water purification systems, medical kits, and communication tools. Identify gaps in your resources and prioritize these in your survival plan.

For instance, if you find that your food supplies are limited, consider what non-perishable items you can stock that are nutrient-dense and easy to prepare. Similarly, evaluate your water purification methods—do you have the necessary filters or purification tablets to ensure access to safe drinking water in an emergency?

Establishing a Survival Strategy

Once you have a comprehensive understanding of risks, needs, and resources, begin developing a detailed survival strategy. This strategy should encompass several key elements:

1. Shelter: Identify a safe location in your home or community where you can take refuge from radiation. This could be a basement or an interior room with minimal windows. If building a dedicated fallout shelter, ensure it is stocked with necessary supplies and can be easily accessed.

2. Stockpiling Essentials: Create a list of essential items to stockpile. Aim for a minimum of two weeks' worth of supplies—food, water, medical supplies, hygiene products, and any special items for family members.

3. Communication: Establish a communication plan that includes a list of emergency contacts, strategies for staying informed, and methods for connecting with loved ones. Consider keeping a battery-operated radio for updates in case of power outages.

4. Evacuation Routes: Identify potential evacuation routes and safe locations outside your immediate area. Familiarize yourself with local geography and have a plan for how you would leave your home if necessary.

5. Regular Review and Drills: Finally, your survival plan should not be static. Regularly review and update it based on changing circumstances or new information. Conduct drills with your household to ensure everyone understands their roles and responsibilities in the event of an emergency.

In conclusion, assessing risks and needs is the foundation of a robust survival strategy. By understanding your unique situation and preparing accordingly, you can enhance your resilience and increase your chances of thriving in a post-nuclear world.

Stockpiling Essentials: Food, Water, and Medicine

In the face of a nuclear threat, preparation is paramount, and a well-thought-out stockpile of essentials can mean the difference between survival and despair. This section outlines crucial considerations for stockpiling food, water, and medicine—three pillars of survival.

Water: The Most Vital Resource

Water is essential for life, and in a post-nuclear scenario, clean water may become scarce. It is generally recommended to store at least one gallon of water per person per day. For a family of four, this translates to 28 gallons for one week. However, considering the potential for prolonged scenarios, aiming for a two-week supply or more is prudent.

Water can be stored in food-grade plastic containers, which are preferable to glass due to their durability. Additionally, purchasing commercially bottled water can serve as a convenient option. It's crucial to rotate your water supply every six months to ensure freshness. If tap water is your primary source, consider investing in water purification tablets or filters capable of removing contaminants and pathogens.

Food: Nutritional and Caloric Needs

When stockpiling food, prioritize items that are non-perishable, nutrient-dense, and easy to prepare. A balanced diet is vital for maintaining physical and mental health, especially under stress. Here are key categories to consider:

1. Grains: Store staples like rice, pasta, and oats. These items have a long shelf life and provide essential carbohydrates. Aim for 25-30 pounds of grains per person for a week.

2. Canned Goods: Canned vegetables, fruits, and proteins (like beans, tuna, or chicken) offer variety and essential nutrients. Each person should ideally have 14-16 cans of protein and vegetables for a week.

3. Dried Foods: Consider dried fruits, nuts, and legumes for snacking and added nutrition. A diverse range will keep morale high and provide essential fats and vitamins. Plan for 5-10 pounds of dried foods per person.

4. Emergency Meals: There are ready-to-eat meals specifically designed for emergencies, such as freeze-dried or dehydrated meals. These can be a practical choice for quick preparation, requiring only water to rehydrate.

5. Cooking Essentials: Don't forget cooking oils, spices, and baking supplies. A small stash of sugar or honey can be comforting and useful for flavoring.

Medicine: Preparing for Health Needs
Medical supplies are often overlooked but are crucial for survival in a crisis. Stock a first aid kit that includes:

- Adhesive bandages, sterile gauze, and tape
- Antiseptic wipes and antibiotic ointment
- Pain relievers (like ibuprofen or acetaminophen)
- Allergy medications, if necessary
- Medication for chronic conditions (enough supply for at least a month)
- A thermometer, scissors, and tweezers

In addition, consider storing supplies to address potential radiation exposure, such as potassium iodide, which can help protect the thyroid gland from radioactive iodine.

Final Considerations
While the above guidelines provide a solid foundation for stockpiling essentials, personal needs and dietary restrictions must also be considered. Regularly review and update your supplies, ensuring items are within their expiry dates and that you have enough for each family member's requirements.

Stockpiling is not just about quantity but also about quality. Aim for a variety of foods to maintain morale and nutrition. Remember, preparation is an ongoing process—stay informed, adapt your supplies based on current events, and engage in community discussions about preparedness. By taking these steps, you can enhance your resilience and ensure that you and your loved ones are better equipped to face the challenges of a post-nuclear world.

Creating a Safe Shelter: DIY Fallout Rooms
In the event of a nuclear explosion, one of the most critical steps for survival is finding or creating a safe shelter that can protect against the immediate and long-term dangers of radiation. Building or adapting a fallout room is an essential part of preparing for such an eventuality. This guide will provide you with the information needed to create a safe space in your home.

Understanding Fallout Protection

Fallout refers to radioactive particles that descend to the ground after a nuclear explosion. These particles can remain hazardous for extended periods, making it imperative to have a shelter that can shield you from radiation. The effectiveness of your fallout room will largely depend on its construction materials, location, and the amount of shielding you can provide.

Location Selection

The ideal location for a fallout room is in the basement or interior of your home, away from windows and external walls. If a basement is not available, choose a central room on the lowest floor possible, such as a bathroom, closet, or pantry. The more concrete, brick, or earth that separates you from the outside, the better your protection against radiation.

Construction Materials

To enhance the shielding capabilities of your fallout room, consider the following materials:

1. Concrete and Brick: These materials are dense and provide excellent radiation shielding. If you are building a room, using reinforced concrete blocks can offer robust protection.

2. Earth and Sandbags: If additional shielding is needed, create a barrier using earth or sandbags. In fact, a layer of dirt or sand can add significant protection, so consider piling it against the walls of your shelter.

3. Lead or Steel: If available, lead sheets or steel can be added to the walls for enhanced radiation protection. However, these materials can be expensive and may not be readily available.

Room Design and Setup

1. Sealing the Room: Ensure that your fallout room is airtight. Use weather stripping and caulk to seal windows and doors. Consider using plastic sheeting to cover any openings and prevent contaminated air from entering.

2. Ventilation: While it's important to seal the room, you also need a way to ventilate it without letting radiation in. Create a makeshift air filtration system using HEPA filters and fans, or consider using an air pump with a one-way valve to allow air in while keeping contaminants out.

3. Supplies and Essentials: Stock your fallout room with essential supplies. This includes non-perishable food, water (at least one gallon per person per day for at least three days), first aid kits, medication, and radiation detection devices. It's also wise to include a battery-operated radio for updates and a manual can opener.

4. Comfort and Hygiene: To ensure that you can stay in the shelter for an extended period, consider the comfort factor. Bring sleeping bags, pillows, and even games or books to help pass the time. For hygiene, include sanitation supplies such as a portable toilet, waste bags, and hand sanitizers.

Psychological Preparedness

Creating a fallout room is not just about physical protection; psychological preparedness is equally important. Understand that being confined in a shelter can induce stress or anxiety. Prepare mentally by discussing plans with family members and establishing a routine once in the shelter. Encourage open communication and support among those inside to foster a sense of community and resilience.

Conclusion

Building a DIY fallout room requires thoughtful planning and preparation. By selecting the right location, utilizing effective materials, and ensuring adequate supplies and comfort, you can significantly enhance your chances of surviving a nuclear event. Remember, preparedness is key to resilience, so take the time to create a safe space that will provide peace of mind in uncertain times.

Communication Plans: Staying Connected with Loved Ones

In the aftermath of a nuclear event, effective communication becomes a cornerstone of survival and resilience. Maintaining contact with loved ones not only provides emotional support but also facilitates critical information exchange about safety, resources, and recovery efforts. Here, we explore practical strategies for establishing robust communication plans to stay connected during and after a nuclear crisis.

1. Establishing Communication Protocols

Before a crisis occurs, families and friends should create a communication protocol that outlines how they will reach each other during emergencies. This protocol should include:

- Primary and Secondary Contacts: Designate a primary contact person outside the immediate area who can relay messages among separated family members. This "communication hub" should be someone who is not directly affected by the nuclear event and can help coordinate information.

- Meeting Points: Identify specific locations where family members can regroup if communication fails. These "safe zones" should be easily accessible and known to all family members.

- Communication Tools: Discuss which devices will be used to communicate, such as cell phones, two-way radios, or even walkie-talkies. Depending on the severity of the situation, some devices may be more reliable than others. Understanding the limitations of technology in a nuclear scenario, where infrastructure may be compromised, is crucial.

2. Utilizing Multiple Communication Channels

In the days following a nuclear event, traditional communication networks may be disrupted. Therefore, utilizing various channels increases the likelihood of staying connected:

- Radio Communication: Battery-operated radios can serve as vital tools for receiving updates from local authorities. Encourage family members to have a portable radio on hand to listen to emergency broadcasts, which can provide critical information about safety protocols and recovery efforts.

- Social Media and Messaging Apps: While mobile networks may be unreliable, internet-based communication platforms can sometimes function if local power sources are intact. Encourage family members to check in via social media or messaging apps, but remain mindful of potential misinformation.

- Emergency Broadcasting Systems: Be aware of local emergency broadcasting systems that may provide instructions and information regarding safety measures, evacuation routes, and resource distribution centers.

3. Developing a Check-In System

Establishing a regular check-in routine can help ease anxiety and ensure everyone is safe. This system can include:

- Scheduled Messages: If communication channels allow, set specific times for family members to check in with one another. This can be as simple as sending a text message or making a brief phone call to confirm safety.

- Code Words: Use pre-arranged code words or phrases that can indicate safety or distress, allowing family members to communicate vital information succinctly.

4. Educating Family Members on Communication Techniques

Ensure that all family members, including children, understand how to use the communication tools available to them. This education should include:

- **Basic Operation of Devices:** Teach family members how to operate radios, cell phones, and other communication devices, including how to recharge them if power sources are available.

- **Emergency Procedures:** Provide guidance on what to do if they cannot reach someone or if they receive concerning information about loved ones. Encourage them to remain calm and follow the established communication protocol.

5. Adapting to Changing Circumstances

In a post-nuclear world, circumstances can change rapidly. Families must remain flexible and ready to adapt their communication plans based on the evolving situation. Regularly review and update communication strategies to account for new developments, ensuring everyone is aware of any changes.

Conclusion

Establishing a solid communication plan before a nuclear event can significantly enhance the chances of staying connected with loved ones during a crisis. By preparing for various scenarios, utilizing multiple communication channels, and ensuring that all members are educated on the procedures, families can navigate the uncertainty of a nuclear crisis with greater resilience and cohesion.

Mental and Emotional Preparedness

In the face of a nuclear crisis, mental and emotional preparedness is as vital as physical readiness. The psychological impact of a nuclear event can be profound, leading to feelings of fear, anxiety, and hopelessness. However, by adopting effective strategies, individuals can cultivate resilience and maintain a sense of calm during such tumultuous times.

Understanding the Psychological Landscape

Before diving into strategies, it's essential to understand the factors that contribute to psychological distress in a nuclear crisis. The unpredictability of nuclear events, coupled with the potential for widespread devastation, can trigger intense anxiety and fear. Acknowledging these feelings is the first step toward managing them. Recognizing that such emotions are normal responses to abnormal situations allows individuals to validate their experiences and prepares them for proactive coping mechanisms.

Developing a Resilience Mindset

1. Fostering a Positive Outlook: Cultivating a resilient mindset starts with focusing on what can be controlled. Maintaining a positive outlook can significantly influence one's emotional response. Engage in positive self-talk, reminding yourself of past challenges you've overcome. This helps to reinforce a belief in your ability to cope with adversity.

2. Setting Realistic Goals: In a crisis, overwhelming situations can lead to paralysis. Setting small, achievable goals can provide a sense of purpose and direction. Whether it's creating a survival plan or establishing a communication network, accomplishing these tasks can instill confidence and reduce anxiety.

3. Practicing Mindfulness and Stress Reduction Techniques: Mindfulness practices, such as meditation and deep-breathing exercises, can help ground individuals in the present moment. These techniques promote relaxation and allow for a clearer mindset amidst chaos. Regular practice of mindfulness can create a buffer against stress and enhance emotional stability.

Building a Support Network

4. Establishing Communication Channels: Maintaining connections with family, friends, and community members is crucial. In times of crisis, having a reliable support network can alleviate feelings of isolation and despair. Create a communication plan to ensure you can reach loved ones, share information, and provide mutual support. Regular check-ins can foster a sense of community, which is vital for emotional well-being.

5. Participating in Community Preparedness: Engaging in community readiness initiatives can offer a sense of belonging and purpose. Working together with others to develop survival strategies and resources can strengthen bonds and provide reassurance. Community collaboration often leads to shared knowledge and resources, enhancing overall preparedness.

Coping with Trauma

6. Understanding the Impact of Trauma: Be aware that trauma responses can manifest in various forms, including anxiety, depression, and post-traumatic stress. Recognizing these symptoms early can help in seeking appropriate support. It's important to normalize these feelings and understand they may arise in the aftermath of a nuclear event.

7. Seeking Professional Help: If feelings of distress become overwhelming, consider reaching out to mental health professionals. Telehealth services may provide accessible support during crises. Professional guidance can aid in developing coping strategies tailored to individual needs.

Emphasizing Routine and Normalcy

8. Establishing Daily Routines: In the aftermath of a nuclear crisis, returning to a semblance of normalcy can be beneficial for mental health. Establishing daily routines, even in a changed environment, can provide structure and predictability. Incorporate activities that promote physical and emotional health, such as exercise, reading, or hobbies.

9. Engaging in Creative Outlets: Expressing emotions through creative outlets such as writing, art, or music can be therapeutic. These activities can serve as healthy coping mechanisms, allowing individuals to process their experiences and emotions constructively.

Conclusion
Mental and emotional preparedness is crucial for navigating the uncertainties of a nuclear crisis. By fostering resilience, establishing support networks, and prioritizing self-care, individuals can maintain emotional well-being even in the face of profound challenges. The strategies outlined above not only help in coping with immediate crises but also lay a foundation for long-term recovery and adaptation in a post-nuclear world.

Chapter 4

During the Attack

Recognizing the Warning Signs

In an era marked by geopolitical tensions and the proliferation of nuclear weapons, understanding the early warning signs of a nuclear strike is paramount for survival. Recognizing these signs can mean the difference between life and death, allowing individuals and communities to take immediate action to protect themselves and their loved ones.

Understanding the Context

Nuclear threats may arise from various sources, including state actors with nuclear capabilities, rogue states, or terrorist organizations. The likelihood of a nuclear event often hinges on escalating political tensions, military maneuvers, and public threats made by leaders. Therefore, keeping abreast of global news and understanding the geopolitical landscape is crucial.

Key Warning Indicators

1. Increased Military Activity: One of the most significant precursors to a potential nuclear strike is a surge in military readiness or unusual military activities. This includes troop mobilizations, military exercises, or the deployment of nuclear-capable missiles. Monitoring defense-related news can provide insights into these developments.

2. Heightened Rhetoric and Threats: Governments may issue aggressive statements or threats regarding nuclear capabilities. Pay attention to public speeches by political leaders, particularly those from countries known to possess nuclear arsenals. Heightened rhetoric can indicate an escalating situation that may lead to conflict.

3. Intelligence Alerts: National intelligence agencies continuously monitor threats and provide alerts to the public. Stay informed through reputable news outlets, government announcements, and official social media channels. If intelligence agencies indicate a heightened threat level, take it seriously.

4. Notification Systems: Many countries have emergency alert systems that notify citizens of imminent threats. These systems may include text alerts, sirens, or broadcasts. Familiarize yourself with these systems and ensure your devices are set up to receive notifications. Regularly check for updates from local authorities.

5. Unusual Environmental Signs: Although rare, certain environmental cues may signal a nuclear event. For example, if you notice a significant increase in air traffic, particularly military aircraft, or if you see unusual movements of military vehicles, these could be preliminary signs of an impending strike.

6. Cybersecurity Threats: In today's digital age, cyberattacks can also be a precursor to a physical strike. Increased cyber activity, especially targeting critical infrastructure, may indicate preparation for a larger action. Stay informed about cybersecurity threats and take precautions to protect your information.

Immediate Response Actions
Upon recognizing potential warning signs, it is essential to respond swiftly and effectively:

1. Seek Shelter: If an imminent threat is confirmed, your first action should be to find a secure shelter. Ideally, this should be a designated fallout shelter or an interior room in your home, away from windows. If no shelter is available, seek underground spaces if possible.

2. Stay Informed: Use radios or other reliable communication devices to listen for updates from authorities. Official channels will provide crucial information on the nature of the threat and instructions on what to do next.

3. Prepare for Impact: Have an emergency kit ready with essentials such as food, water, medications, a flashlight, and a first-aid kit. This kit should be easily accessible in your designated shelter.

4. Communicate with Loved Ones: Establish a communication plan with family and friends. Knowing how to reach each other in the event of a strike will help alleviate anxiety and ensure that everyone is accounted for.

5. Remain Calm and Rational: Panic can lead to poor decisions. Focus on the facts, trust your preparation, and act according to your plan. Keeping a clear mind will help you navigate the situation more effectively.

Conclusion
Recognizing the warning signs of a nuclear strike is a critical skill in today's world. By staying informed and prepared, you can enhance your chances of survival in the face of one of humanity's gravest threats. Awareness and preparedness are your best defenses against the unimaginable.

Seeking Immediate Shelter: The Golden Hour

In the event of a nuclear explosion, the critical window of time known as the "Golden Hour" represents the first hour following the detonation. During this period, the actions taken by individuals can significantly influence their chances of survival. Finding immediate shelter is vital, and understanding why this is critical, as well as how to effectively seek shelter, can mean the difference between life and death.

Why Finding Shelter Quickly is Critical

1. Blast Wave Impact: A nuclear explosion generates an immense blast wave that can obliterate structures within a wide radius. This wave travels at supersonic speeds, causing destructive winds that can uproot trees, shatter windows, and collapse buildings. The closer one is to ground zero, the more urgent the need for shelter is, as the immediate vicinity can be lethal.

2. Thermal Radiation: The explosion produces an intense flash of thermal radiation, resulting in severe burns and igniting fires within seconds. Individuals exposed to this radiation can suffer third-degree burns or worse, depending on their distance from the blast. Seeking shelter can significantly reduce the risk of exposure to this immediate and deadly heat.

3. Nuclear Fallout: After the initial explosion, radioactive particles are propelled into the atmosphere and can settle over a large area, contaminating air, water, and food supplies. Fallout can begin to descend within minutes, making immediate sheltering essential to minimize exposure. The longer one remains outside, the higher the risk of inhaling or coming into contact with these dangerous particles.

4. Psychological Safety: The chaos and destruction following an explosion can be overwhelming. Finding shelter not only protects from physical harm but also provides a sense of security and psychological relief amidst the panic. Establishing a safe space allows individuals to gather their thoughts, assess their situation, and make more informed decisions.

How to Seek Shelter Effectively

1. Know Your Options: Before an event occurs, familiarize yourself with potential shelter locations. The best options include basements, underground parking garages, or any well-constructed building. If these are unavailable, seek out interior rooms on the lowest floors, preferably without windows.

2. Act Quickly: When a nuclear detonation occurs, time is of the essence. Do not waste precious moments assessing the situation or gathering unnecessary belongings. Instead, move swiftly toward the nearest shelter, ideally within a minute or two of the blast.

3. Seal the Shelter: Once you've reached a safe location, take immediate steps to seal it off from outside air. Close windows, doors, and vents to minimize the intake of radioactive particles. Use duct tape or other materials to cover any gaps that might allow contaminated air to enter.

4. Stay Informed: If possible, bring a battery-operated radio or a charged mobile device to receive updates on the situation. Authorities will provide information about the hazards of fallout, when it is safe to exit the shelter, and guidance on next steps.

5. Prepare for an Extended Stay: While the immediate focus is on seeking shelter, it is important to be mentally prepared for the possibility of remaining in the shelter for an extended period. Ensure you have essential supplies such as food, water, and medical equipment, and establish a system for rationing these resources.

In conclusion, the Golden Hour following a nuclear explosion is a critical time for survival. By understanding the urgency of finding immediate shelter and knowing how to act promptly, individuals increase their chances of overcoming the initial threats posed by a nuclear event and can better secure their safety in the ensuing chaos.

Protecting Yourself from Radiation

In the event of a nuclear explosion, radiation exposure poses one of the most significant threats to survival. Understanding how to protect yourself from radiation is crucial for minimizing health risks. This section outlines effective techniques to safeguard against radiation exposure in the aftermath of a nuclear incident.

1. Seek Immediate Shelter

The urgency of finding shelter cannot be overstated. In the first moments following a nuclear detonation, the primary concern should be to locate a secure place that can shield you from both the blast and subsequent radiation. Ideally, this shelter should be constructed of dense materials—such as concrete, brick, or earth—which can effectively block radiation. Basements or interior rooms of buildings, away from windows, provide better protection than those closer to the outside.

2. Seal Your Shelter

Once you have found a suitable shelter, it is essential to seal it off from outside air and potential fallout. Use duct tape and plastic sheeting to cover windows, doors, and vents to prevent radioactive particles from entering. If your shelter has access to an air supply, consider using air filters—if available—to further reduce contamination. The goal is to create a barrier that minimizes the influx of radioactive dust and particles.

3. Stay Indoors
Remaining indoors is one of the most effective means of reducing radiation exposure. The radiation intensity decreases significantly with distance from the source, and staying inside can drastically limit your exposure to radioactive fallout. The principle of 'time, distance, and shielding' applies here: by staying away from the area of immediate danger and using the building materials around you as shielding, you can reduce the radiation dose you receive.

4. Monitor Radiation Levels
If you have access to a radiation detector, use it to monitor radiation levels in and around your shelter. Understanding the radiation environment will help you make informed decisions about when it is safe to leave your shelter. In the absence of a Geiger counter or similar device, remain informed through emergency broadcasts if available, as authorities will provide updates about radiation levels and safe evacuation times.

5. Limit Time Outside
If you must venture outside—whether to gather supplies or check on loved ones—limit your time spent in the open air. Quick trips can minimize radiation exposure; aim to stay outside for as little time as possible. When you do go outside, wear protective clothing such as long sleeves, pants, gloves, and a mask to reduce skin exposure and inhalation of radioactive particles.

6. Decontamination Procedures
Should you come into contact with radioactive materials, follow decontamination procedures diligently. Remove any clothing that may have been contaminated and seal it in a plastic bag. Wash your skin thoroughly with soap and water to remove any particles. If you have access to a decontamination station, take advantage of it. Remember that it is crucial to avoid spreading contamination to your shelter.

7. Stay Informed
Keeping up-to-date with information from local authorities will help you make better decisions regarding your safety. Listen to emergency radio broadcasts or use battery-operated devices to receive alerts about changing radiation conditions and recommendations for evacuation or sheltering.

Conclusion
Protecting yourself from radiation involves a proactive approach that prioritizes immediate shelter, sealing off your environment, and minimizing exposure time. By understanding and implementing these techniques, you can significantly reduce the risks associated with radiation

exposure in the aftermath of a nuclear event. Your survival depends not only on your actions but also on your ability to remain calm, informed, and prepared.

Communicating with Authorities and Loved Ones

In the aftermath of a nuclear event, effective communication becomes a lifeline for survival, enabling individuals to stay informed about the evolving situation, receive crucial instructions from authorities, and maintain connections with loved ones. Understanding the tools available for communication and the strategies to employ them is essential for enhancing safety and resilience in a chaotic environment.

1. Establishing Communication Channels

In the immediate aftermath of a nuclear explosion, conventional communication systems (such as cell phones and internet services) may become unreliable or entirely inoperable due to damage, overload, or electromagnetic interference from the blast. Therefore, it is vital to have alternative methods prepared in advance:

- **Battery-Powered Radios:** A battery-operated AM/FM radio can keep you informed about emergency broadcasts and updates from local authorities. Look for models that can also receive shortwave frequencies, which may provide information from a broader range of sources.

- **Two-Way Radios:** Walkie-talkies or ham radios can facilitate communication among family members and close community networks when traditional systems fail. These radios can operate over various distances and are less likely to be affected by external disruptions.

- **Emergency Communication Apps:** In situations where the internet remains available, apps like WhatsApp, Signal, or Telegram can provide messaging services even when cellular networks are down, as they rely on internet connectivity. Ensure these apps are downloaded and functional before an emergency arises.

2. Creating a Communication Plan

Preparation is key to effective communication. Families should develop a comprehensive communication plan that includes:

- **Designated Meeting Points:** Identify safe locations where family members can regroup if separated. This could be a neighbor's house, a local community center, or a designated shelter.

- **Emergency Contacts:** Compile a list of important contact numbers, including extended family, friends, and emergency services. Distribute this list to all family members. Consider designating an out-of-area contact whom everyone can reach in case local communication becomes compromised.

- Regular Check-In Times: Establish specific times for family members to check in with each other if they are separated. This routine can provide structure and reassurance during a crisis.

3. Staying Informed and Trusting Sources
In a post-nuclear environment, misinformation can spread rapidly, complicating decision-making and increasing panic. **To combat this:**

- Verify Information: Always cross-check information from multiple reliable sources before acting on it. Government channels, local emergency management agencies, and established news organizations are typically trustworthy sources.

- Listen for Official Messages: Tune into emergency broadcasts on radio stations or follow updates from official government social media accounts to receive the latest directives regarding safety, evacuation routes, and resource distribution.

4. Utilizing Community Networks
Building and relying on community networks can enhance communication and support during times of crisis:

- Community Meetings: Participate in local preparedness meetings before a crisis occurs. Establishing relationships with neighbors can facilitate better communication during emergencies.

- Neighborhood Watch Programs: Engage in or create community safety initiatives that enhance communication and coordination in response to threats, including nuclear attacks.

- Social Media Groups: Join community-based groups on social media platforms that can serve as information hubs during an emergency. These groups can facilitate the sharing of resources, updates, and support among members.

Conclusion
In the face of a nuclear disaster, communication is vital for survival and recovery. By preparing in advance, utilizing a variety of communication tools, and fostering community connections, individuals can enhance their ability to stay informed and maintain contact with loved ones. This proactive approach will not only aid in immediate survival but also lay the groundwork for rebuilding and reconnecting in the aftermath of a catastrophic event.

Staying Safe Indoors: Sealing Your Shelter
In the event of a nuclear explosion, the immediate danger does not end with the blast itself; the fallout that follows poses a significant threat to life and health. Therefore, ensuring that your

shelter is properly sealed against radioactive particles is crucial for survival. This section outlines practical steps to enhance your shelter's security against fallout.

1. Identify the Shelter Location
Your shelter should ideally be located underground or in the center of your home, away from windows and exterior walls. The further you are from the outside, the better your protection from radiation. If constructing a new shelter, choose a site that is naturally shielded by earth or other materials.

2. Seal All Openings
To minimize the entry of radioactive particles, it is vital to seal all openings in your shelter:

- **Windows and Doors:** Use plastic sheeting, duct tape, or weather stripping to cover windows and doors. Ensure that all gaps are tightly sealed to prevent air infiltration. If you have a basement, consider sealing off windows and using heavy furniture to block potential entry points.

- **Vents and Ducts:** Close off ventilation systems. Use filters designed to block particles, or if unavailable, seal vents with duct tape and plastic sheeting. Ensure that any exhaust fans or air ducts are turned off to prevent fallout from being drawn into your shelter.

- **Cracks and Crevices:** Inspect the shelter for any cracks or crevices in walls, floors, and ceilings. Use caulk or expanding foam to fill these gaps. Pay special attention to areas around electrical outlets, plumbing fixtures, and any other penetrations in the structure.

3. Create a Decontamination Zone
Set up an area outside your main living space where individuals can decontaminate upon entering. This can be a small enclosed space or a designated area inside the shelter. **Equip it with:**

- **Plastic Sheeting:** Line the area with plastic sheeting to catch any fallout that may be brushed off.

- **Supplies:** Keep supplies like soap, water, and towels for cleaning skin and clothes. Have a container for contaminated clothing and items that need to be disposed of safely.

4. Air Filtration Systems
If possible, invest in a high-efficiency particulate air (HEPA) filter or an air purifier equipped with a HEPA filter. These can significantly reduce airborne radioactive particles. Make sure to keep the air circulating but through filtered paths to limit exposure.

5. Stockpile Essential Supplies

While ensuring the structure is sealed, also consider what you'll need to survive comfortably within it. Stock up on:

- Food and Water: Non-perishable foods and enough water to last for several weeks. Remember, radiation can contaminate external water sources, so having a supply is vital.

- Emergency Kits: Include first aid supplies, flashlights, batteries, and a battery-operated radio for updates.

6. Communications Setup

Establish a communication plan with loved ones outside your shelter. Ensure you have a battery-powered or hand-crank radio to receive news and updates. If possible, have a means of communication that does not rely on external power sources, as infrastructure may be compromised.

7. Regular Checks and Maintenance

Regularly inspect your shelter to ensure that it remains sealed and that supplies are adequate. Rotate food and medical supplies to prevent expiration, and check the integrity of the shelter's sealing mechanisms.

Conclusion

Sealing your shelter against nuclear fallout is a critical step toward ensuring your survival in the aftermath of a nuclear explosion. By taking proactive measures to secure your environment, you can significantly reduce your risk of radiation exposure and enhance your chances of staying safe until it is deemed safe to emerge. Remember, preparedness is key, and a well-thought-out plan can make all the difference in a crisis.

Chapter 5

The First 24 Hours After a Nuclear Explosion

Assessing the Situation: Understanding the Damage

In the immediate aftermath of a nuclear explosion, understanding the extent of the damage is crucial for survival and recovery. The assessment process must be systematic, focusing on both physical destruction and human impact. Here, we outline key considerations and steps for evaluating the situation in the wake of a nuclear event.

1. Initial Safety Checks

Before venturing out to assess damage, ensure your immediate environment is safe. If you are in a shelter, remain there until you have verified that it is safe to exit. Look for signs of structural integrity: listen for creaks, observe for cracks in walls, and check for any signs of compromised stability. Ensuring your safety first can prevent further injury.

2. Immediate Surroundings

Once it is safe to exit, start by surveying your immediate surroundings. Look for the following indicators of destruction:

- **Blast Damage:** Identify anything that has been destroyed or severely damaged due to the blast wave. This includes buildings, trees, and infrastructure such as power lines and roads. Understanding the destruction radius of the explosion can help gauge how far the impact extends.

- **Thermal Damage:** Assess areas for signs of fire or severe burns. Thermal radiation can ignite fires that spread rapidly, and understanding fire hazards in your vicinity is essential for safety.

- **Radiation Exposure:** Use any available radiation detection devices to ascertain radiation levels. This is crucial, as radiation can remain hazardous long after the explosion. If radiation is detected, assess how it may affect your immediate area and your ability to move safely.

3. Evaluating Casualties

If you come across others, check for injuries or casualties. The psychological toll of witnessing destruction and suffering can be immense. Approach individuals cautiously, as panic and shock can cause unpredictable behavior. Provide first aid to those in need if you are trained, and prioritize those with life-threatening injuries.

4. Understanding Fallout

Nuclear fallout consists of radioactive particles that can contaminate the environment. It is essential to understand the pattern of fallout distribution, which can be influenced by wind and weather conditions. Use any available information regarding the prevailing winds at the time of the explosion to estimate which areas may be more contaminated. Avoid these areas as much as possible.

5. Resource Assessment

Evaluate your available resources, including water, food, and medical supplies. In a post-nuclear environment, access to clean water may be severely compromised, so prioritize locating and securing safe water sources. Take inventory of food supplies and begin rationing if necessary to extend your provisions.

6. Communication and Information Gathering

Establish a means of communication with others. Use radios or other communication devices to gather information about the broader situation. Understanding the extent of the disaster beyond your immediate area is critical for making informed decisions about evacuation or seeking aid.

7. Long-Term Considerations

As you assess the immediate damage, begin considering long-term survival strategies. This includes planning for shelter, food, and water sources in a potentially altered environment. Assess the feasibility of relocating to safer areas and the implications of longer-term exposure to radiation.

Conclusion

Assessing the situation after a nuclear explosion is a multi-faceted process that requires careful evaluation of immediate risks, available resources, and the health and safety of those around you. By approaching the assessment methodically, you can develop a more comprehensive understanding of the damage and make informed decisions that enhance your chances of survival in a profoundly changed world.

Managing Water and Food Supplies

In the immediate aftermath of a nuclear explosion, managing water and food supplies becomes one of the most critical aspects of survival. The choices made within the first hours can significantly impact the ability to endure the ensuing days and weeks. Understanding how to prioritize these essential resources can mean the difference between survival and succumbing to the harsh realities of a post-nuclear environment.

Assessing Available Resources

The first step in managing water and food supplies is to conduct a thorough assessment of what is available. Identify all potential sources of potable water, such as stored bottled water, water in pipes, and any reservoirs or natural sources nearby, such as lakes or rivers. However, it's crucial to remember that water from these natural sources may be contaminated due to fallout. Therefore, prioritize stored water until it can be tested or treated.

For food, inventory any supplies you have on hand. This includes canned goods, dried foods, and any perishable items that may be salvageable. If you are in a shelter, check for food that can be stored long-term, which is often canned or vacuum-sealed products. Avoid consuming any food from compromised sources, such as areas exposed to fallout.

Prioritizing Water Needs

Water is essential for hydration, sanitation, and cooking. In the initial hours post-explosion, your primary focus should be on conserving water, as access to clean water may be limited. The average person needs at least one gallon of water per day for drinking and sanitation, but in a crisis, rationing becomes crucial.

1. Establish a Rationing Plan: Start by determining how much water you have and dividing it into manageable portions. Aim to limit consumption to about half a gallon per person per day, if necessary, while prioritizing hydration over other uses.

2. Purification Techniques: If you must use unknown water sources, familiarize yourself with purification methods. Boiling water for at least one minute can kill most pathogens, and if you have access to purification tablets or filters, use them.

3. Collecting Rainwater: In a longer-term situation, consider collecting rainwater using tarps or containers. This can provide a sustainable source of water, but be cautious of contamination from fallout or debris.

Maximizing Food Supplies

Food supplies will also dwindle quickly in a crisis, so it is essential to manage what you have wisely. Focus on calorie-dense foods that provide maximum energy with minimal volume, such as nuts, granola bars, and dried fruits.

1. Rationing Food: Just as with water, food should be rationed. Begin by distributing smaller portions to everyone, ensuring that all individuals receive a fair share without depleting stocks too quickly.

2. Utilizing Perishables: If you have access to perishable items, consume them first. This includes dairy products, meats, and fruits that can spoil quickly. Cooking or preserving these items can extend their usability.

3. Food Preparation: In a survival situation, efficiency matters. Prepare meals that require minimal energy and resources. Focus on cooking methods that do not require extensive fuel or equipment, such as boiling or using a simple camp stove.

4. Foraging and Hunting: As time progresses, consider foraging for edible plants or hunting small game if it is safe to do so. Familiarize yourself with local flora and fauna prior to any crisis to ensure you can identify safe food sources.

Emotional Considerations
Managing water and food supplies is not just a logistical challenge but also an emotional one. Anxiety about scarcity can lead to panic, so it is essential to maintain a calm demeanor and work collaboratively with others to prioritize and ration resources effectively. Establishing a routine for resource management can also help instill a sense of normalcy in an otherwise chaotic environment.

In conclusion, prioritizing water and food supplies in the immediate aftermath of a nuclear explosion is vital for survival. By assessing available resources, rationing effectively, and employing purification methods, survivors can navigate the challenging initial hours and set the foundation for their long-term survival.

Addressing Injuries and Health Concerns
In the chaotic aftermath of a nuclear explosion, the immediate priority is the health and safety of oneself and others. In addition to the physical destruction caused by the blast, survivors face a myriad of injuries and health concerns exacerbated by the presence of radiation. Understanding basic first aid and the specifics of managing radiation sickness can be crucial for survival in this dire situation.

Basic First Aid for Common Injuries
First aid is essential in the immediate hours following a nuclear event. Survivors may encounter injuries ranging from cuts and bruises to more severe traumas. Here are some foundational first aid techniques:

1. Assessing the Scene: Before providing assistance, ensure your safety and that of the injured individual. Look for ongoing hazards, such as unstable structures or additional explosions.

2. Wounds and Bleeding: For cuts and abrasions, clean the wound with clean water and, if available, mild soap. Apply a sterile dressing or clean cloth and secure it with tape or a bandage. For severe bleeding, apply direct pressure to the wound with a clean cloth or bandage until the bleeding stops. If possible, elevate the injured body part above heart level to slow the bleeding.

3. Burns: Burns may occur from the thermal blast or subsequent fires. Cool the burn with lukewarm (not cold) water for at least 10 minutes. Cover the burn with a sterile, non-stick dressing. Avoid using ice, butter, or ointments, as these can worsen the injury.

4. Fractures and Sprains: If a fracture is suspected, immobilize the injured area using splints made from available materials (e.g., wood, cardboard). Apply ice packs wrapped in cloth to reduce swelling, but avoid direct contact with the skin.

5. Shock: Signs of shock include pale skin, rapid pulse, and confusion. Lay the person down, elevate their legs, and keep them warm with blankets or clothing. Do not give them food or drink if they are unconscious or semi-conscious.

Managing Radiation Sickness

Radiation sickness occurs when an individual is exposed to high levels of radiation, particularly from fallout. Symptoms can manifest within hours or days and may include nausea, vomiting, fatigue, and hair loss. Here's how to manage it:

1. Recognize Symptoms: Be vigilant for symptoms of radiation sickness, which can range from mild to severe. Early symptoms may include nausea, vomiting, diarrhea, and fatigue. As exposure severity increases, symptoms may escalate to confusion, fever, and bleeding.

2. Decontamination: If you suspect exposure, decontaminate as quickly as possible. Remove contaminated clothing and wash skin thoroughly with soap and water to eliminate radioactive particles. If water is limited, brushing off dust and debris can help reduce contamination.

3. Hydration and Nutrition: Maintaining hydration is crucial. If clean water is available, encourage fluid intake to help flush out toxins. In cases of nausea, small sips might be more manageable. If food is accessible, focus on bland foods that can be easier on the stomach, but avoid anything that could worsen nausea.

4. Seek Medical Attention: While immediate medical care may be challenging, keep a lookout for any signs of severe radiation sickness. If professionals are available, they may provide treatments such as potassium iodide to protect the thyroid from radioactive iodine, or other interventions specific to radiation exposure.

5. Monitoring Health: Establish a system for monitoring the health of those affected by radiation. Keep track of symptoms, and when circumstances allow, seek medical attention for advanced treatments, especially for individuals exhibiting severe symptoms or those who were closer to the blast.

Conclusion
In the aftermath of a nuclear explosion, understanding basic first aid and the management of radiation sickness can dramatically increase the chances of survival. By remaining calm, assessing injuries, and applying effective first aid techniques, individuals can mitigate health risks while waiting for further assistance. It is vital to prepare for these scenarios, as the ability to respond effectively can make a significant difference in a life-threatening situation.

Dealing with Psychological Trauma
In the aftermath of a nuclear explosion, the psychological impact can be as devastating as the physical destruction. Survivors may experience intense feelings of shock, fear, grief, and helplessness. Understanding how to cope with these emotions is crucial for mental health and resilience. This section outlines effective strategies for dealing with psychological trauma in a post-nuclear environment.

Acknowledge Your Feelings
The first step in coping with psychological trauma is acknowledging your feelings and experiences. It's normal to feel a wide range of emotions, including fear, anger, confusion, and despair. Allow yourself to express these feelings, whether through talking, journaling, or other forms of emotional release. Suppressing emotions can lead to increased stress and mental health issues, so give yourself permission to feel and process what has happened.

Establish a Routine
Creating a daily routine can provide a sense of normalcy and stability amidst chaos. Structure helps to mitigate feelings of uncertainty and helplessness. Include basic tasks such as meal preparation, hygiene, and shelter maintenance in your daily schedule. Simple routines can instill a sense of control over your environment, which is vital for mental well-being during traumatic times.

Connect with Others
Social support is essential for emotional healing. Reach out to family members, friends, or community members who have also experienced the trauma. Sharing your experiences and feelings with others who understand can foster a sense of belonging and decrease feelings of

isolation. If in-person connections are not possible, consider using communication tools, like radios or other devices, to maintain contact. Establishing support networks can provide emotional sustenance and practical assistance in navigating the aftermath.

Practice Mindfulness and Relaxation Techniques

Mindfulness and relaxation techniques can significantly reduce stress and anxiety. Practices such as deep breathing exercises, meditation, and yoga can help ground you in the present moment, alleviating overwhelming feelings of fear and anxiety. Spend a few minutes each day focusing on your breath or engaging in gentle movements to promote relaxation and emotional regulation.

Focus on Basic Self-Care

Physical health is closely tied to mental health, especially in the aftermath of a crisis. Ensure that you are eating nutritious foods, drinking enough water, and getting adequate rest. Engage in physical activity or light exercise, which can release endorphins and improve mood. Basic self-care practices can bolster your resilience against psychological trauma.

Seek Professional Help When Possible

While immediate access to mental health professionals may be limited in a post-nuclear environment, look for opportunities to connect with mental health resources when available. If you feel comfortable, seek out individuals who are trained in psychological first aid or trauma response to guide you through your feelings. Professional help can provide valuable coping strategies and support for trauma recovery.

Engage in Creative Expression

Creative expression can serve as a powerful outlet for processing trauma. Engage in activities such as drawing, writing, or music to express your thoughts and feelings. Creative practices can facilitate emotional processing, help to make sense of experiences, and foster a sense of agency in your recovery.

Limit Exposure to Distressing News

In times of crisis, the constant barrage of distressing news can exacerbate feelings of anxiety and trauma. While it is crucial to stay informed, limit your exposure to news and media that may trigger negative emotions. Set specific times to check updates and focus on reliable sources to avoid misinformation.

Conclusion

Dealing with psychological trauma after a nuclear event is a challenging but manageable process. By acknowledging your feelings, establishing routines, connecting with others, practicing self-care, and utilizing coping strategies, you can foster resilience in the face of unimaginable adversity. Remember that healing is a journey, and it is essential to be patient and compassionate with yourself as you navigate the complexities of trauma recovery.

Understanding and Monitoring Radiation Levels

In the aftermath of a nuclear explosion, assessing radiation levels becomes crucial for survival. Understanding how to monitor radiation effectively can help individuals make informed decisions about their safety and the safety of their loved ones. This section will explore the types of radiation detectors available, how to use them, and critical considerations for determining when it is safe to move from a shelter.

Types of Radiation Detectors

1. Geiger-Müller (GM) Counters: The most common type of radiation detector, GM counters measure alpha, beta, and gamma radiation. They provide real-time readings and audible clicks or beeps to indicate the presence of radiation. GM counters are portable and relatively easy to use, making them suitable for personal safety monitoring.

2. Scintillation Counters: These detectors use a special material that emits light (scintillation) when it interacts with radiation. Scintillation counters are highly sensitive and can detect low levels of radiation, making them ideal for assessing contamination on surfaces.

3. Dosimeters: Personal dosimeters are small devices worn on clothing that measure an individual's cumulative exposure to radiation over time. They are essential for monitoring exposure levels during prolonged periods in contaminated environments.

4. Radiation Survey Meters: These devices are used for more extensive area monitoring and can quantify the radiation levels in specific locations. They are essential for determining safe paths for movement and identifying contaminated zones.

How to Use Radiation Detectors

Using radiation detectors effectively involves a few key steps:

1. Familiarization: Before a nuclear event occurs, familiarize yourself with your radiation detection equipment. Understand how to operate it, interpret the readings, and calibrate it if necessary.

2. Location Monitoring: After a nuclear explosion, begin monitoring the area surrounding your shelter. Move slowly and methodically, taking measurements at different distances and angles to ensure a comprehensive assessment of radiation levels.

3. Interpreting Readings: Radiation levels are typically measured in microsieverts per hour (µSv/h). It's important to familiarize yourself with baseline readings for your area, which can help you understand what constitutes a significant increase in radiation. For example, levels above 0.1 µSv/h may warrant caution, while readings above 1 µSv/h indicate a higher risk.

4. Assessing Contamination: Use scintillation counters for surface contamination checks, particularly on clothing, skin, and shelter surfaces. If the detector indicates elevated levels on surfaces, take precautions to limit exposure.

When It's Safe to Move

Determining when it is safe to leave your shelter is a critical decision that should be made based on the following considerations:

1. Radiation Levels: If radiation levels are significantly reduced to below the threshold of concern (ideally under 0.1 µSv/h), it may be safe to venture outside. However, assessing the environment and potential hazards is essential before making this decision.

2. Time Factor: The intensity of radiation decreases over time due to the decay of radioactive isotopes. The "golden hour" immediately following a blast is crucial; exposure should be minimized during this time, as radiation levels can be at their highest. Over the course of days and weeks, levels may decrease significantly.

3. Emergency Alerts: Pay attention to communication from local authorities through radios or other communication devices. These alerts can provide updates on radiation levels and guidance on evacuation or movement.

4. Personal Safety Measures: When deciding to move, ensure you are equipped with protective clothing, such as masks and coveralls, to minimize radiation exposure. Use your detector to monitor levels continuously as you navigate outside.

In summary, understanding and monitoring radiation levels is paramount for survival in a post-nuclear environment. By utilizing appropriate detection devices, interpreting readings accurately, and making informed decisions about movement, individuals can protect themselves from the dangers of radiation exposure.

Chapter 6

Surviving the First Week

Maintaining Your Shelter

In the aftermath of a nuclear explosion, maintaining a secure and livable shelter is crucial for survival. The conditions within your shelter can determine your overall health and safety, making daily routines and systematic checks essential for long-term survival. Here's a comprehensive guide on how to establish and maintain an effective routine to keep your shelter secure and livable.

1. Daily Inspections

Every day, conduct a thorough inspection of your shelter. Pay attention to the structural integrity of the walls, ceiling, and entrances. Look for any signs of damage from blast waves or subsequent settling. Check for leaks or breaches that could allow radioactive fallout or contaminants to enter. If you notice any deterioration, prioritize repairs immediately to ensure the shelter remains secure.

2. Ventilation Management

Proper ventilation is critical, especially in a confined space. Monitor the air quality inside your shelter regularly. Ensure that your ventilation systems—whether they involve air filters or manual openings—are functioning properly. If you have sealed your shelter to minimize external contamination, it might be necessary to create a controlled airflow to avoid buildup of harmful gases. Always have backup systems in place, such as battery-operated fans or hand-cranked devices, to maintain airflow.

3. Radiation Monitoring

Equip your shelter with radiation detection tools, such as Geiger counters or dosimeters. Check radiation levels daily to assess safety. Understanding the levels of radiation is vital to determine when it might be safe to venture outside or if further sealing measures are necessary. Keep track of the readings in a log to identify patterns or changes in radiation levels over time.

4. Resource Management

Establish a routine for resource management, focusing on food and water supplies. Regularly check the condition of your food and water stockpiles. Rotate supplies to ensure nothing expires or degrades. Ration your resources according to a set schedule, taking daily inventory of what you have consumed and what remains. This practice not only prolongs your supplies but also helps you plan for future needs.

5. Sanitation Protocols
Maintaining hygiene is vital to prevent the spread of disease in a confined environment. Establish daily sanitation routines, including waste management practices. Designate areas for waste disposal, and ensure that these areas are kept clean and contained. Use approved methods for decontamination of surfaces and personal items. Regularly wash your hands and ensure that any food preparation areas are sanitized to minimize health risks.

6. Communication Checks
In a post-nuclear scenario, staying informed is critical. Allocate time each day to check your communication devices—radios, satellite phones, or any other means of receiving updates from the outside world. Establish a schedule for listening to broadcasts and set aside periods for trying to contact loved ones or local networks. This will help maintain a sense of connection to the outside world and ensure you are informed about ongoing conditions.

7. Mental and Emotional Care
The psychological impact of living in a post-nuclear environment can be profound. Incorporate daily routines that promote mental well-being. This could include scheduled times for relaxation, meditation, or group discussions if sheltering with others. Create a space within your shelter that is dedicated to these activities, which can help alleviate stress, foster community, and enhance morale.

8. Emergency Drills
Lastly, conduct regular emergency drills to ensure that everyone in your shelter knows what to do in case of a sudden crisis. Practice evacuation procedures, radiation exposure protocols, and communication plans. These drills reinforce preparedness and can significantly reduce panic in a real emergency situation.

By adhering to these daily routines and checks, you can maintain a secure and livable shelter during a nuclear crisis, enhancing your chances of survival while fostering a sense of stability and community among those you shelter with.

Resource Management
In the aftermath of a nuclear event, the ability to manage and ration food and water becomes critical for survival. With the potential for long-term disruptions to supply chains and environmental contamination, understanding effective rationing strategies can be the

difference between life and death. Here are key considerations and strategies for extending your supplies.

Understanding Your Supplies

First and foremost, assess what you have on hand. Take inventory of all food and water sources. This includes packaged goods, canned items, dried foods, and any existing water supplies. Understanding the nutritional content and shelf life of your supplies is crucial. Prioritize items that are calorie-dense and nutrient-rich, as they will provide the necessary energy and sustenance while minimizing consumption.

Establishing Rationing Guidelines

Once you have a clear picture of your supplies, establish a rationing plan. The goal is to extend your resources while maintaining health and energy levels. Here are some guidelines to consider:

1. Caloric Needs: Assess the caloric needs of each individual in your shelter. An average adult requires approximately 2,000 to 2,500 calories per day under normal circumstances. In survival situations, particularly in the aftermath of a nuclear event, physical activity may vary. Adjust portions accordingly; a reduced caloric intake of around 1,500 to 2,000 calories per day may suffice to maintain energy levels while preserving resources.

2. Food Rationing: Create daily rations based on your inventory. For example, if you have 30 cans of food and plan to survive for 15 days, distribute the food evenly to ensure each person has enough to eat throughout that period. Consider diversifying the types of food consumed to maintain morale and avoid dietary deficiencies. Incorporate protein sources, carbohydrates, and fats in your rations, if possible.

3. Water Rationing: Water is even more critical than food in a survival scenario. An average adult requires about 2 liters (or half a gallon) of water per day under normal conditions. In a crisis, aim to ration water to about 1 liter per person per day, reserving more for critical needs such as hydration after physical exertion or for medical emergencies. Use water sparingly for cooking, cleaning, and personal hygiene.

Techniques to Extend Supplies

1. Minimize Waste: Be vigilant about avoiding waste. Use leftover food creatively, turning scraps into new meals, or incorporating all parts of vegetables when possible. Store food properly to prevent spoilage and protect it from contamination.

2. Purification Techniques: If water supplies dwindle, learn purification methods to make non-potable water safe for consumption. Boiling water, using water purification tablets, or employing filtration systems can help extend your water supply. Always have a backup plan for sourcing water, such as collecting rainwater or locating potential sources nearby.

3. Consider Foraging: Depending on the environment, foraging for edible plants, mushrooms, and wild fruits can supplement your food supply. However, ensure you have knowledge about foraging to avoid toxic plants.

4. Gardening: If time and conditions allow, consider establishing a small garden or container plants that can yield food. Fast-growing crops such as radishes, lettuce, and herbs can provide some nutrition if conditions permit.

Monitoring and Adapting

Regularly monitor your supplies and adjust your rationing plan as needed. Keep a close eye on the remaining food and water, and be prepared to adapt your strategies based on the changing circumstances. Effective communication among shelter inhabitants about resource management will foster a sense of community and shared responsibility.

In conclusion, effective resource management through careful rationing of food and water can significantly enhance your chances of survival in a post-nuclear event. By planning, monitoring, and adapting your strategies, you can extend your supplies and navigate the challenges that arise in such a crisis.

Staying Informed: Gathering News and Updates

In the aftermath of a nuclear event, reliable information becomes a vital resource for survival and recovery. The chaos and uncertainty that follow such a catastrophe can lead to misinformation, panic, and confusion. Therefore, understanding how to gather news and updates from trustworthy sources is crucial for making informed decisions that can affect your safety and wellbeing.

Understanding Information Sources

Reliable information sources can be divided into two main categories: official sources and independent media. Official sources include government agencies, emergency management organizations, and international bodies like the World Health Organization (WHO) and the International Atomic Energy Agency (IAEA). These organizations often provide real-time updates on safety protocols, radiation levels, and resource availability.

On the other hand, independent media outlets can also serve as valuable resources, provided they adhere to journalistic standards and fact-checking. It's essential to vet any media source for credibility and reliability by looking for long-standing reputations, editorial standards, and transparency in reporting.

Establishing a Communication Network

In a post-nuclear world, communication infrastructures may be severely disrupted. Establishing a communication network within your community can be instrumental in sharing updates and coordinating responses. Consider forming small groups with neighbors or trusted individuals where information can be exchanged. This community network can help disseminate reliable news and combat misinformation.

Utilizing tools such as two-way radios or ham radios can also facilitate communication when traditional networks fail. These devices can connect you with local emergency services or other community members, providing an alternative means to receive updates.

Utilizing Technology Wisely

While technology can be a boon for gathering information, it also comes with risks, especially regarding misinformation. Prior to any nuclear event, familiarize yourself with reliable apps and websites that can provide accurate information. Government websites, reputable news outlets, and specialized emergency management apps can be critical in times of crisis.

In addition, social media platforms can be a double-edged sword. While they can offer immediate updates, they are also platforms for the rapid spread of rumors. If using social media, follow verified accounts of reputable organizations and journalists. Look for posts that cite official sources, and be wary of unverified claims that can incite panic or lead to poor decision-making.

Critical Thinking and Information Verification

In a highly charged environment, critical thinking becomes paramount. When you receive news updates, consider the following questions:

1. Who is the source? Check the credentials and track record of the source. Is it a recognized authority in emergency management or public health?

2. What is the evidence? Are the claims supported by data or reports? Look for references to studies, official statements, or corroborating evidence.

3. Why is the information being shared? Analyze the intent behind the news. Is it to inform, incite fear, or persuade action? Understanding the motivation can help you gauge the reliability of the information.

4. What do other sources say? Cross-reference the information with multiple credible sources. If the same news is reported across several reputable outlets, it is more likely to be accurate.

Conclusion

In a post-nuclear context, staying informed is not just about gathering news; it's about ensuring that the information you receive is reliable and actionable. By establishing a communication network, utilizing technology wisely, and applying critical thinking, you can navigate the uncertainty that follows a nuclear event, make informed decisions, and ultimately protect yourself and your community. Remember, in times of crisis, accurate information can be as vital as food, water, and shelter.

Hygiene and Sanitation in a Confined Space

In the aftermath of a nuclear explosion, maintaining hygiene and sanitation within a confined space is crucial for survival. The immediate environment is likely to be fraught with challenges, including limited resources, the potential for contamination, and the psychological toll of confinement. Proper hygiene and sanitation practices can help prevent illness, promote mental well-being, and sustain overall health amid the chaos.

1. Understanding the Importance of Hygiene

In a post-nuclear scenario, the risk of infectious diseases rises significantly due to compromised living conditions. Contaminated water, limited access to medical care, and increased stress levels can lead to a range of health issues. Maintaining good hygiene practices helps to reduce the risk of infections and illnesses, ensuring that individuals and families remain as healthy as possible.

2. Waste Management

Effective waste management is one of the most critical aspects of sanitation in confined spaces. Human waste can be a significant source of disease if not handled properly. Here are some strategies for managing waste:

- **Designate a Waste Area:** If possible, create a specific area for waste disposal, away from living quarters and food storage. This area should be clearly marked and should not be disturbed.

- Use Containers: Use sealed containers for human waste. Depending on your resources, this could be a portable toilet, a bucket with a tight-fitting lid, or even a plastic bag. Make sure to line containers with plastic bags for easier disposal.

- Regular Disposal: Plan for regular disposal of waste. If you can safely do so, bury the waste at a distance from your shelter, at least 200 feet away, to minimize contamination risk. Follow local guidelines for waste disposal if available.

- Biodegradable Options: If you have access to biodegradable waste bags, consider using them for easier decomposition and less environmental impact.

3. Hand Hygiene
Proper hand hygiene is vital to preventing the spread of germs and infections. Here are practical steps to maintain hand hygiene:

- Handwashing: Use soap and clean water whenever available. If water is scarce, use hand sanitizer with at least 60% alcohol content. Establish a routine for handwashing, especially after using the toilet and before handling food.

- Moist Towelettes: In situations where running water is unavailable, keep a stash of moist towelettes or alcohol wipes handy for cleaning hands.

- Avoid Touching Face: Encourage all members of the group to avoid touching their faces, particularly the eyes, nose, and mouth, as this can facilitate the entry of pathogens.

4. Food Hygiene
Food safety should be a top priority to prevent foodborne illnesses. Follow these guidelines to maintain food hygiene:

- Storage: Store food in airtight containers to protect against contamination and pests. Keep perishable items in a cool, dry place.

- Preparation: Wash hands before preparing any food. If possible, use clean utensils and surfaces. If you have limited cleaning resources, wipe surfaces with a clean cloth before use.

- Cooking: Whenever possible, cook food thoroughly to kill any pathogens. Use safe methods for heating food, and avoid eating raw or undercooked items.

5. Mental Health and Sanitation

Maintaining hygiene and sanitation is not merely a physical necessity; it also plays a crucial role in mental health. A clean environment can foster a sense of control and normalcy in a chaotic situation. Encourage routines that involve cleaning and organizing the shelter as a way to boost morale and create a sense of community among those in confinement.

Conclusion

In a confined space following a nuclear event, hygiene and sanitation become paramount for survival. By implementing effective waste management, promoting hand hygiene, ensuring food safety, and fostering a clean environment, individuals can significantly reduce health risks and enhance their chances of survival. Maintaining these practices will not only protect physical health but also contribute to the mental well-being of everyone involved, making it imperative to prioritize hygiene in this challenging context.

Planning for the Long-Term: What Comes Next?

In the aftermath of a nuclear event, the first week can be characterized by chaos, uncertainty, and the instinctual drive to survive. However, as the immediate danger begins to subside, it becomes crucial to transition from short-term survival strategies to long-term planning. Understanding your situation and preparing for life beyond the initial crisis is essential for ensuring not only physical survival but also emotional and psychological well-being.

Assessing Your Situation

The first step in long-term planning involves a thorough assessment of your immediate surroundings and resources. Begin by evaluating the safety of your shelter. Look for signs of structural damage, contamination, or radiation levels that could compromise your safety. Utilize any available radiation detection tools to measure ambient radiation, and remain indoors until you are certain it is safe to venture outside.

Next, assess your supplies: food, water, medical resources, and essential tools. Inventory what you have on hand and determine how long these supplies will last under current consumption rates. This assessment will guide your rationing strategies and highlight the need for sustainable sourcing in the days to come.

Understanding the broader environment is also critical. This includes identifying potential hazards—such as contamination zones or areas with active conflict—and determining safe routes for future travel. Familiarize yourself with the local geography and any pre-existing community resources that might be available, such as farms or water sources.

Establishing a Sustainable Routine

Once you have assessed your situation, establishing a sustainable daily routine will help restore a sense of normalcy and control. This routine should include tasks such as food gathering, sanitation, security checks, and community engagement. Regularity in daily activities can provide psychological stability during a time of upheaval.

Incorporate resource management techniques into your routine. Learn how to ration food and water effectively, ensuring that you can extend your supplies as long as possible. Create a system for rotating perishable items and regularly check your stored supplies for spoilage.

Moreover, hygiene and sanitation must be prioritized to prevent illness. Develop waste management practices and ensure that any water used for drinking or cooking is purified, as contaminated sources can pose significant health risks.

Seeking Community Support

Isolation can exacerbate feelings of fear and anxiety, making it essential to seek out community support. If you are part of a local network, engage with neighbors and community members to share resources, skills, and information. Collaborative efforts can enhance survival strategies, such as pooling supplies, sharing knowledge about safe foraging, and providing mutual aid in medical care.

Consider forming or joining a community group focused on long-term recovery. This network can develop plans for rebuilding infrastructure, restoring security, and sharing responsibilities for resource management. A strong community can serve as a lifeline, providing emotional support and practical assistance.

Planning for the Future

As you stabilize your immediate survival situation, begin to contemplate longer-term goals. This may include plans for sustainable living, such as growing food, finding clean water sources, and establishing a secure and habitable environment. Research and learn new skills related to agriculture, hunting, and gathering, as well as basic medical care and first aid.

Additionally, consider the psychological aspects of long-term survival. Engage in practices that promote mental resilience, such as mindfulness, meditation, or community gatherings that foster social connections. This emotional preparedness will be essential as you navigate the challenges of life in a post-nuclear world.

In conclusion, transitioning from immediate survival to long-term planning is a critical step in the aftermath of a nuclear disaster. By assessing your situation, establishing sustainable routines, seeking community support, and planning for the future, you can not only survive but also begin to rebuild and thrive in a drastically changed environment.

Chapter 7

Long-Term Survival Strategies

Finding Safe Water Sources

In the aftermath of a nuclear event, securing safe water sources is one of the most critical survival priorities. Water can become contaminated due to radioactive fallout, chemical pollutants, or disruption of water supply systems. Here's how to locate, test, and purify water effectively to ensure your health and safety in a post-nuclear environment.

Locating Water Sources

1. Natural Sources: Start by searching for natural water sources, such as rivers, streams, lakes, and ponds. These are often the most accessible sources of water. However, it's essential to remember that these sources may be contaminated, especially in the wake of a nuclear incident.

2. Rainwater Collection: Collecting rainwater is another viable option. Use clean containers to gather rainwater, ensuring that the collection area is free from debris that could contaminate the water. Rainwater is typically safer than surface water, but it should still be purified before consumption.

3. Groundwater: If you have access to a hand pump or can dig a well, groundwater can be a relatively clean source. However, it is crucial to be cautious, as groundwater can also be contaminated by radioactive substances leaching into the soil.

4. Urban Areas: In urban settings, check for water from building systems, such as hot water tanks, toilet tanks, and even swimming pools. While these sources may be less contaminated than open water bodies, they still require purification.

Testing Water for Contamination

Before consuming water, testing its safety is vital. Here are some methods for testing water:

1. Simple Visual Inspection: Look for signs of contamination such as unusual color, cloudiness, or floating debris. If the water appears discolored or has an odd odor, it's best to avoid using it.

2. Chemical Test Kits: Invest in portable water testing kits, which can detect the presence of common contaminants, including bacteria, heavy metals, and radiation. These kits are often used for testing water quality in emergency situations.

3. Radiation Detectors: Use Geiger counters or other radiation detection devices to measure the level of radioactivity in the water. If radiation levels exceed safe thresholds, do not consume the water.

Purifying Water

Once you have located a potential water source and tested it, the next step is purification. Here are some effective methods:

1. Boiling: Boiling water for at least one minute (or three minutes at higher altitudes) is one of the most reliable methods of purification. This process kills bacteria, viruses, and parasites. However, boiling does not remove chemical contaminants or radioactive particles.

2. Filtration: Use water filters designed to remove pathogens. Look for filters that can also remove heavy metals and chemical contaminants. While many household filters may not be effective against radiation, specialized filters exist for this purpose.

3. Chemicals: Water purification tablets, often containing iodine or chlorine dioxide, can disinfect water effectively. Follow the instructions carefully, as the dosage depends on the water's clarity and volume.

4. Solar Purification: If sunlight is available, consider using solar stills. This method utilizes the sun's heat to evaporate water, which then condenses on a surface and can be collected as purified water. While slow, it is effective for removing many contaminants, including salt and some chemicals.

5. Activated Charcoal: After filtering or boiling, running water through activated charcoal can enhance purification by removing impurities and improving taste.

Final Thoughts

In a post-nuclear environment, finding and ensuring safe water sources is paramount for survival. By effectively locating water, testing for contaminants, and employing purification methods, individuals can significantly reduce health risks and increase their chances of long-term survival. Preparation and knowledge are essential, so familiarize yourself with these techniques ahead of time to bolster your resilience in a crisis.

Growing and Sourcing Food Post-Attack

In the aftermath of a nuclear attack, food security becomes a critical concern as existing food supplies may be contaminated or inaccessible. Re-establishing sustainable food production and foraging strategies is essential for survival in a post-nuclear world. This section outlines practical techniques for growing food and sourcing it in a contaminated environment.

1. Understanding Soil Contamination

Before beginning any growing efforts, it's crucial to assess the level of soil contamination. Nuclear fallout can introduce radioactive isotopes into the soil, which can be harmful if ingested by plants. Conduct soil tests if possible, using available kits to measure radiation levels. Avoid planting in areas with high contamination. If contamination is suspected but not confirmed, consider using raised beds or containers filled with uncontaminated soil.

2. Container Gardening

Container gardening provides a viable option for growing food in potentially contaminated areas. Utilizing pots, buckets, or any available containers, you can create a controlled environment for your plants. Ensure that the growing medium is free from contaminants by sourcing soil from safe areas or using commercially available organic potting mixes. Container gardening also allows you to move plants to areas with better sunlight or protection from adverse weather.

3. Hydroponics and Aquaponics

Hydroponics, the method of growing plants in nutrient-rich water, can be an effective way to produce food without soil. This system is particularly useful in urban environments or areas where soil is heavily contaminated. Similarly, aquaponics combines fish farming with hydroponics, creating a symbiotic environment where fish waste provides nutrients for the plants, while the plants help filter the water for the fish. Both methods require careful management of water quality and nutrient levels but can lead to efficient food production.

4. Foraging for Wild Edibles

In the absence of cultivated crops, foraging for wild edibles can supplement your diet. Knowledge of local flora is essential, as many plants can provide nutrition. Start by learning to identify safe and edible plants, such as dandelions, wild garlic, and various berries. However, caution is paramount; avoid areas that are likely to be contaminated and ensure that you can accurately identify plants to avoid toxic varieties. Field guides or local experts can assist with plant identification.

5. Permaculture Techniques

Implementing permaculture principles can help create a self-sustaining food system. This includes designing your garden layout to maximize the use of space and resources. Techniques such as companion planting—growing mutually beneficial plants together—can enhance biodiversity and promote pest resistance. Incorporating methods like mulching, composting, and rainwater harvesting can also improve soil health and water availability, creating a more resilient food production system.

6. Livestock and Insect Farming

If conditions allow, consider small-scale livestock farming. Chickens, rabbits, and goats can provide critical sources of protein and other resources. Chickens, for example, can lay eggs, while rabbits reproduce quickly and require minimal space. Insect farming, particularly crickets and mealworms, is another sustainable protein source that requires less space and resources than traditional livestock.

7. Preservation Techniques

Effective food preservation methods will extend the life of your harvests. Techniques such as dehydrating, canning, and fermenting can help you store surplus food for future use. Understanding these methods not only reduces waste but also allows for better management of available resources over time.

Conclusion

In a post-nuclear world, food production and sourcing will heavily rely on creativity, resourcefulness, and knowledge of sustainable practices. By understanding soil safety, utilizing container gardening, exploring foraging options, applying permaculture techniques, raising small livestock, and mastering food preservation, individuals and communities can work towards achieving food security amidst challenging conditions. The ability to produce and source food sustainably will be pivotal in rebuilding lives and communities after a nuclear event.

Establishing a New Normal: Daily Life After a Nuclear War

The aftermath of a nuclear war presents a stark and daunting reality for survivors. The devastation of infrastructure, loss of life, and pervasive fear of radiation create an environment that is fundamentally different from the world that existed prior to the attack. Establishing a new normal in this drastically altered landscape requires resilience, adaptability, and a commitment to rebuilding both individual lives and communities.

Understanding the New Landscape

In the wake of a nuclear attack, the immediate environment will be fraught with challenges. Urban areas may be uninhabitable due to destruction and contamination, while rural regions might offer safer locales but lack resources and infrastructure. Survivors will need to assess their surroundings carefully, identifying safe zones and potential hazards such as radiation hotspots or contaminated water sources. Developing skills in environmental assessment becomes crucial; learning to use radiation detectors and understanding how to interpret their readings will aid in navigating this new world.

Daily Routines: Structure and Stability

Creating a daily routine can provide a sense of normalcy amid chaos. Survivors should prioritize basic needs such as food, water, and shelter while establishing consistent daily practices. Routines might include gathering and purifying water, foraging for edible plants, and tending to any gardens or crops grown in safe soil. Regularly scheduled check-ins with community members can bolster morale and foster a sense of cooperation.

Physical health will be paramount in the new normal. Developing hygiene practices, even in resource-scarce environments, is critical to prevent the spread of disease. Daily routines should incorporate methods for managing waste, cleaning contaminated surfaces, and maintaining personal cleanliness to safeguard against illness.

Community Collaboration: The Cornerstone of Survival

In a post-nuclear world, the importance of community cannot be overstated. Establishing a network of support among survivors will not only provide practical benefits, such as shared resources and labor, but will also address the psychological need for connection and collective resilience. Regular community meetings can serve as platforms for sharing knowledge, distributing resources, and coordinating efforts for rebuilding.

Community collaboration may extend to creating communal gardens, establishing security protocols, and organizing barter systems for food and supplies. Empowering individuals to take on roles based on their skills—be it farming, medical care, or engineering—can enhance the group's overall capability to thrive in this new normal.

Adapting Skills and Knowledge

Survivors must embrace a mindset of continuous learning and adaptation. Many modern conveniences will be lost, necessitating the revival of traditional skills. Knowledge in areas such as agriculture, hunting, foraging, and basic construction becomes invaluable. Communities should prioritize skill-sharing workshops where individuals can teach and learn from one another, ensuring that essential skills are preserved and passed on.

Mental health support is equally important in establishing a new normal. The trauma of surviving a nuclear war can be profound, leading to anxiety, depression, and post-traumatic stress. Encouraging open discussions about mental health and finding ways to support one another through shared experiences can foster resilience. Engaging in community-building activities, storytelling, and shared rituals can offer emotional healing and strengthen social bonds.

Fostering Hope and Resilience

Finally, survivors must cultivate hope and resilience. This involves focusing on the possibility of rebuilding rather than merely surviving. Setting tangible goals, whether related to food production, infrastructure repair, or community cohesion, can instill a sense of purpose. Encouraging creativity and innovation in problem-solving will inspire individuals to envision a better future, emphasizing that the new normal, although different, can be an opportunity for growth and rejuvenation.

In conclusion, establishing a new normal after a nuclear war is a multifaceted challenge that requires adaptation, community collaboration, and a focus on rebuilding with hope. By harnessing collective strengths, sharing knowledge, and nurturing emotional well-being, survivors can navigate the complexities of this transformed world and lay the groundwork for a resilient future.

Staying Healthy

In the aftermath of a nuclear event, the healthcare landscape is drastically altered, presenting unique challenges for survivors. Conventional medical facilities may be compromised or entirely unavailable, necessitating a shift toward self-reliance and resourcefulness in managing health. This section outlines practical strategies for preventing disease and injury in a post-nuclear world, emphasizing the importance of hygiene, nutrition, injury management, and community support.

1. Hygiene Practices

Maintaining proper hygiene is paramount to preventing illness in a resource-limited environment. Without access to running water or sanitation facilities, survivors must adapt their practices:

- **Water Purification:** Always ensure that any water sourced is purified before consumption. Techniques such as boiling, using water purification tablets, or filtering through cloth can eliminate many pathogens. Establish a routine for boiling water whenever possible.

- **Hand Hygiene:** Encourage regular hand washing with available resources. If soap is scarce, using ash or sand as a scrub can be effective. Always wash hands before eating, after using the restroom, and after handling waste.

- **Waste Management:** Establish designated areas for human waste disposal, away from food and water sources. This can include digging latrines or using a bucket system lined with bags to minimize contamination. Ensure waste is covered and disposed of safely to prevent disease transmission.

2. Nutrition and Food Safety

A balanced diet is critical for maintaining health, especially during high-stress scenarios. While food sources may be limited, focus on the following:

- **Foraging and Farming:** Identify local edible plants and potential sources of food. Knowledge of foraging can yield fruits, nuts, and greens that are safe to consume. Consider establishing small gardens using any viable seeds available to supplement nutrition.

- **Preserving Food:** With limited refrigeration, develop techniques for preserving food such as drying, smoking, or canning. Stockpile non-perishable items when possible, and rotate supplies to prevent spoilage.

- **Nutritional Balance:** Aim for a diet rich in vitamins and minerals. If possible, prioritize foods high in protein and fiber to support energy levels and overall health.

3. Injury Management

In the absence of modern medical facilities, treating injuries effectively is crucial:

- **Basic First Aid:** Equip yourself with knowledge of first aid for common injuries such as cuts, burns, fractures, and sprains. In the absence of sterile bandages, clean cloth can be used to cover wounds. Regularly check for signs of infection, including redness, swelling, and pus.

- **Burn Treatment:** For burns, cool the area with clean, cool water for at least 10 minutes. Cover the burn with a non-stick dressing or clean cloth. Avoid breaking blisters, as this can lead to infection.

- Handling Chronic Conditions: Individuals with chronic health issues should develop plans for managing their conditions. This may involve natural remedies or alternative treatments, such as herbal medicines, which can help alleviate symptoms in the absence of pharmaceuticals.

4. Community Health Support

Collaboration and mutual support within communities can significantly enhance health outcomes:

- Skill Sharing: Encourage community members with medical knowledge to share their skills. Organize workshops on basic first aid, herbal medicine, and nutrition to empower others.

- Resource Pooling: Establish a community resource pool for sharing medical supplies, tools, and knowledge. This can enhance the overall resilience and health of the community.

- Mental Health: Recognize the importance of mental well-being. Foster community connections through group activities, discussions, and support networks to help individuals cope with trauma and stress.

In conclusion, staying healthy in a post-nuclear world demands proactive measures focused on hygiene, nutrition, injury management, and community support. By adapting to new realities and fostering a spirit of collaboration, individuals can enhance their resilience and capacity to thrive despite the challenges posed by a drastically changed environment.

Rebuilding and Reconnecting with Society

In the aftermath of a nuclear event, the landscape of society will be dramatically altered. The immediate focus will be on survival: securing food, water, and shelter. However, as basic needs are met, the critical task of rebuilding and reconnecting with society becomes paramount. Community resilience is essential for long-term survival and recovery, and understanding how to foster connections can facilitate a smoother transition into a new normal.

1. Assessing Community Needs and Resources

The first step in rebuilding a community is assessing the existing needs and available resources. Gather those who survived the initial disaster to discuss the community's current situation. This assessment should include:

- Identifying Skills and Talents: Engage community members in sharing their skills, whether in agriculture, construction, medical care, or mechanics. Skills inventories can help determine how best to utilize available human resources.

- Mapping Resources: Identify local resources such as water supplies, arable land, and shelter options. Understanding what is available will help in planning sustainable living arrangements.

2. Establishing Communication Networks

Effective communication is vital for coordination and organization. Establishing a reliable communication network can:

- Facilitate Information Sharing: Create systems for sharing vital information regarding safety, resources, and community activities. Simple methods like bulletin boards, word-of-mouth, and designated meeting times can work effectively in low-tech environments.

- Maintain Morale: Regular gatherings foster a sense of unity and belonging, which is crucial in a post-crisis environment. These meetings can serve as platforms for discussing issues, sharing experiences, and providing emotional support.

3. Creating a Collaborative Governance Structure

As communities begin to stabilize, establishing a governance structure can help maintain order and facilitate decision-making. **This structure should prioritize:**

- Inclusivity: Ensure that all voices are heard in the rebuilding process, especially marginalized groups, to foster a sense of ownership and community solidarity.

- Conflict Resolution: Develop mechanisms for resolving disputes amicably. Clear rules and processes can help prevent conflicts from escalating and promote cooperation.

4. Re-establishing Social Bonds

Rebuilding social connections is essential for emotional recovery and community strength. **Initiatives that can help include:**

- Community Events: Organizing communal activities such as potlucks, skill-sharing workshops, or cultural events can reintegrate members and strengthen ties.

- Support Groups: Forming groups focused on mental health, grief processing, and trauma recovery can provide a safe space for individuals to share their experiences and feelings.

5. Fostering Economic Resilience

Rebuilding the local economy is crucial for long-term survival. **Communities can:**

- Encourage Bartering and Sharing: In the absence of stable currency, establishing systems for bartering goods and services can help meet needs while fostering interdependence.

- **Support Local Agriculture:** Reestablishing food production through community gardens or cooperatives can enhance food security and provide a sense of purpose.

6. Embracing Education and Skill Development

Education will be essential in the rebuilding phase. Communities should:

- **Promote Knowledge Sharing:** Implement informal education systems where individuals can teach one another essential skills—whether practical, technical, or emotional.
- **Adapt to New Realities:** Encourage learning about sustainable practices, such as permaculture, first aid, and self-defense, to empower community members in navigating their new environment.

Conclusion

Rebuilding and reconnecting with society after a nuclear event is a multifaceted process that requires cooperation, empathy, and resilience. By assessing needs, establishing communication networks, creating governance structures, fostering social bonds, enhancing economic resilience, and promoting education, communities can lay the groundwork for a robust recovery. It is through these efforts that individuals will not only survive but thrive, as they forge new connections and rebuild a sense of community in a changed world.

Chapter 8

Radiation: Understanding and Coping

What is Radiation? Types and Effects

Radiation is the energy emitted in the form of particles or electromagnetic waves as a result of nuclear reactions, radioactive decay, or other processes. It can be classified into two primary categories: ionizing and non-ionizing radiation. Understanding these categories is crucial, especially in the context of nuclear warfare and its aftermath, as they have varying effects on human health and the environment.

Ionizing Radiation

Ionizing radiation has enough energy to remove tightly bound electrons from atoms, creating ions. This process can disrupt atomic structures and lead to chemical changes in living cells. The main types of ionizing radiation include:

1. Alpha Particles: Composed of two protons and two neutrons (the equivalent of a helium nucleus), alpha particles are relatively heavy and carry a positive charge. They cannot penetrate human skin but can cause significant damage if ingested or inhaled. Inside the body, alpha emitters can lead to cellular damage and increase the risk of cancer.

2. Beta Particles: These are high-energy, high-speed electrons or positrons emitted during radioactive decay. They can penetrate the skin but are generally stopped by a few millimeters of tissue. Beta radiation can cause skin burns and increase cancer risk, particularly if beta-emitting substances are ingested or inhaled.

3. Gamma Rays: Gamma radiation consists of high-energy electromagnetic waves. Unlike alpha and beta particles, gamma rays have no mass and no charge, allowing them to penetrate most materials, including human tissue. This makes them particularly dangerous during a nuclear explosion and in the case of radioactive contamination, as they can damage internal organs and tissues at a cellular level.

4. Neutrons: Neutron radiation consists of free neutrons released during nuclear reactions. Neutrons can penetrate deeply into materials, including human tissues, and can lead to significant biological damage. Neutron radiation is particularly problematic in nuclear reactors or during nuclear weapon detonations.

Non-Ionizing Radiation

Non-ionizing radiation has less energy than ionizing radiation and is generally considered less harmful. It includes:

1. Ultraviolet (UV) Radiation: While UV radiation can cause skin burns and increase the risk of skin cancer, it does not carry enough energy to ionize atoms directly. However, prolonged exposure can damage the DNA in skin cells, leading to mutations and, eventually, cancer.

2. Electromagnetic Fields (EMFs): EMFs, including radio waves, microwaves, and infrared radiation, are present in various technologies. While some studies suggest potential links to health effects, the consensus is that non-ionizing radiation is significantly less harmful than ionizing radiation.

Health Effects of Radiation Exposure

The health effects of radiation exposure depend on several factors, including the type of radiation, the dose received, the duration of exposure, and the individual's health condition. Acute exposure to high levels of ionizing radiation can lead to:

- **Radiation Sickness:** Symptoms may include nausea, vomiting, fatigue, and skin burns, depending on the dose.
- **Increased Cancer Risk:** Long-term exposure to ionizing radiation increases the likelihood of developing various cancers, particularly leukemia and solid tumors.
- **Genetic Damage:** Radiation can cause mutations in DNA, potentially leading to hereditary health issues in future generations.

In contrast, low-level exposure, such as that which might occur from environmental sources or certain medical treatments, is generally considered safe, although the cumulative effects are still a subject of ongoing research.

In conclusion, radiation encompasses a range of energy emissions with variable effects on human health, particularly in the context of nuclear events. Understanding the types of radiation and their impacts is essential for effective preparedness and response strategies in the event of a nuclear catastrophe.

Radiation Sickness

Radiation sickness, also known as acute radiation syndrome (ARS), occurs when an individual is exposed to a high dose of ionizing radiation over a short period. Understanding the symptoms and treatment options is crucial for anyone facing the possibility of a nuclear event, as timely intervention can significantly affect health outcomes.

Symptoms of Radiation Sickness

The onset of symptoms typically depends on the radiation dose received and can manifest within hours to days following exposure. The primary symptoms fall into three distinct phases:

1. Prodromal Phase: This initial phase may occur within minutes to days after exposure and can last from a few hours to several days. **Common symptoms include:**
- Nausea and vomiting
- Diarrhea
- Fatigue and weakness
- Loss of appetite
- Fever

2. Latent Phase: After the initial symptoms subside, there may be a period of apparent health improvement lasting from a few hours to several weeks. During this time, the severity of symptoms can vary based on the dose of radiation exposure. However, this latency can be deceptive, as it is followed by the more severe effects of radiation damage.

3. Manifest Illness Phase: This phase can be more severe and includes a range of symptoms depending on the body systems affected:

- **Hematopoietic Syndrome (dose of 1-10 Gy):** Affects the bone marrow, leading to a decrease in blood cell production. Symptoms include:
  - Increased susceptibility to infections
  - Bleeding and bruising
  - Anemia
- **Gastrointestinal Syndrome (dose of 6-30 Gy):** Involves damage to the gastrointestinal tract, resulting in:
  - Severe nausea and vomiting
  - Diarrhea
  - Dehydration
- **Cerebral Syndrome (dose above 30 Gy):** A rare but life-threatening condition that affects the central nervous system, leading to:
  - Confusion
  - Loss of consciousness
  - Seizures

Treatment of Radiation Sickness

The treatment of radiation sickness focuses on supportive care, symptom management, and the use of specific medical interventions depending on the severity of the exposure.

1. Immediate Care:

- **Evacuation:** The first step is to remove the affected individual from the radiation exposure area to limit further absorption.
- **Decontamination:** If clothing is contaminated, it should be removed to reduce radiation exposure. Washing the skin with soap and water helps remove radioactive particles.

2. Supportive Treatment:

- **Hydration:** Maintaining fluid intake is vital, especially for those experiencing vomiting and diarrhea. Intravenous (IV) fluids may be necessary for severe cases.
- **Nutritional Support:** Given the potential for gastrointestinal damage, ensuring proper nutrition is essential. This may require enteral or parenteral nutrition.
- **Symptomatic Relief:** Medications can be administered to manage pain, nausea, and vomiting.

3. Specific Treatments:

- **Bone Marrow Treatment:** For individuals with hematopoietic syndrome, treatments such as hematopoietic growth factors (e.g., G-CSF) may be used to stimulate blood cell production.
- **Potassium Iodide:** In cases of radioactive iodine exposure, potassium iodide can be administered to prevent the absorption of iodine by the thyroid gland, thereby reducing cancer risk.
- **Antibiotics and Blood Transfusions:** These may be necessary to treat infections and manage severe anemia.

4. Long-Term Care:

Survivors of radiation sickness may require ongoing medical evaluations to monitor for long-term complications, including cancer and other chronic health issues.

Awareness of radiation sickness symptoms and treatment options can significantly influence survival and recovery outcomes. In a post-nuclear scenario, preparation and immediate action can mitigate the devastating effects of radiation exposure.

Long-Term Health Risks

The detonation of a nuclear weapon releases an overwhelming amount of energy and radiation, resulting in immediate destruction and loss of life. However, the long-term health implications of radiation exposure extend far beyond these initial effects. Understanding these risks is critical for individuals who may find themselves in post-nuclear scenarios, as well as for public health officials and policymakers.

Types of Radiation and Their Impact

Radiation exposure can occur in various forms, including alpha particles, beta particles, and gamma rays, each with distinct characteristics and potential health effects. Alpha particles, though less penetrating, can cause significant damage if ingested or inhaled. Beta particles can penetrate skin and cause burns, while gamma rays, being highly penetrating, can affect internal organs and tissues from a distance. The energy from these radiations can alter cellular structures and DNA, leading to mutations.

Cancer Risks

One of the most significant long-term health effects associated with radiation exposure is an increased risk of cancer. The relationship between radiation exposure and cancer is well-established, with numerous studies indicating that even low doses of radiation can lead to an elevated risk. The risk of developing cancer is influenced by several factors, including the dose of radiation received, the duration of exposure, the age at exposure, and individual genetic susceptibility.

The most common cancers associated with radiation exposure include:

- **Leukemia:** This cancer of the blood-forming tissues is particularly linked to exposure to ionizing radiation, with studies showing a notable increase in cases among survivors of the Hiroshima and Nagasaki bombings.
- **Thyroid Cancer:** Due to the thyroid gland's ability to absorb iodine, it is particularly vulnerable to radioactive iodine isotopes. Increased cases of thyroid cancer have been documented in populations exposed to fallout.
- **Solid Tumors:** Cancers of the breast, lung, and stomach have also been shown to increase following significant radiation exposure. The latency period for these cancers can be extensive, often taking years or even decades to manifest.

Non-Cancerous Health Effects

While cancer is the most well-known consequence of radiation exposure, non-cancerous health effects can also arise. These include:

- **Cataracts:** Radiation exposure can lead to the development of cataracts, which are clouding of the lens in the eye that can impair vision.
- **Cardiovascular Disease:** Some studies suggest a potential link between radiation exposure and an increased risk of heart disease and stroke, although the mechanisms remain less understood compared to cancer.
- **Reproductive Health Issues:** Radiation can affect reproductive health, potentially leading to infertility, miscarriages, or congenital disabilities in future generations.

Monitoring and Mitigation

In a post-nuclear environment, monitoring radiation levels becomes critical for assessing health risks. Individuals and communities should be trained to use radiation detection devices to evaluate exposure levels. Moreover, medical professionals should be equipped to recognize the signs of radiation sickness and the long-term health effects associated with exposure.

Preventive measures, such as regular health check-ups and screenings for those at risk, can aid in early detection of cancers and other diseases. Public health campaigns will be essential to educate affected populations about the symptoms of radiation-related health issues and the importance of seeking timely medical intervention.

Conclusion

The long-term health risks of radiation exposure following a nuclear event are profound and multifaceted, with cancer being the most significant concern. Understanding these risks is crucial for preparedness and recovery efforts in the aftermath of a nuclear catastrophe. Awareness, monitoring, and proactive health measures can help mitigate the long-term effects of radiation exposure and improve the chances of survival and recovery for affected populations.

Reducing Radiation Exposure: Dos and Don'ts

In the aftermath of a nuclear explosion or any radiation-related incident, minimizing radiation exposure becomes paramount for survival and health. Understanding the practical steps you can take to protect yourself and your loved ones is essential. Here's a comprehensive guide of dos and don'ts aimed at helping individuals reduce their exposure to radiation in their daily activities.

Dos

1. Stay Indoors: The most effective way to reduce radiation exposure is to remain indoors, particularly in a well-sealed shelter. Close all windows, doors, and ventilation systems to prevent radioactive fallout from entering. Ideally, stay in the most central room of your home, away from exterior walls.

2. Seal Your Shelter: Use duct tape and plastic sheeting to seal windows and doors. This adds an extra layer of protection against airborne particles. Ensure that any cracks or openings are tightly covered to minimize exposure.

3. Monitor Radiation Levels: If possible, obtain a Geiger counter or radiation detector. Regularly monitor the radiation levels in and around your shelter. This information will help you understand when it is safe to venture outside.

4. Limit Time Outside: If you must go outdoors, minimize the time spent outside. The longer you are exposed to radiation, the greater the risk of harmful effects. Plan your activities to be as quick and efficient as possible.

5. Use Protective Clothing: If you need to go outside, wear long-sleeved clothing, gloves, and a mask. This will help protect your skin and respiratory system from radioactive particles. After returning indoors, remove these clothes carefully to avoid bringing contamination inside.

6. Decontaminate: If you come into contact with potentially radioactive materials, decontaminate yourself immediately. Remove your clothing and shower thoroughly to wash off any particles that may have settled on your skin or hair.

7. Stay Informed: Use a battery-operated radio or other reliable communication methods to stay updated on the situation outside. Follow instructions from local authorities regarding safety measures and evacuation orders.

8. Eat and Drink Cautiously: Consume only pre-packaged food and bottled water that have not been exposed to the environment. Avoid eating fresh produce from local sources until you are certain of its safety.

Don'ts

1. Don't Panic: While the situation may be alarming, keeping a clear mind is crucial. Panic can lead to poor decision-making and increased exposure due to hasty actions.

2. Don't Ignore Official Guidance: Always follow the instructions from emergency services and officials. Ignoring safety protocols can increase your risk of exposure.

3. Don't Use Vacuum Cleaners: Avoid using vacuum cleaners to clean up dust or debris that may be contaminated. This can spread radioactive particles into the air. Instead, use damp cloths to wipe surfaces.

4. Don't Eat or Drink Unverified Sources: Avoid consuming food or water that has been exposed to the outdoors unless it has been properly tested and deemed safe. This includes local water supplies that may be contaminated.

5. Don't Engage in Outdoor Activities: Avoid outdoor activities that can increase your exposure, such as gardening, exercising, or any other non-essential tasks.

6. Don't Forget Hygiene: While it's important to protect yourself from radiation, maintaining hygiene is also crucial. However, avoid using potentially contaminated water for washing. Use bottled water for personal hygiene if necessary.

7. Don't Risk Long-Term Exposure: If you must evacuate, do so only after assessing the radiation levels and understanding the risks. Prolonged exposure to contaminated areas can have serious health implications.

By following these dos and don'ts, individuals can significantly reduce their radiation exposure during and after a nuclear incident. Remember, preparedness and knowledge are your best defenses against radiation risks. Stay informed, stay safe, and prioritize health in uncertain times.

Decontaminating Your Environment

In the aftermath of a nuclear explosion, one of the most critical aspects of ensuring safety and health is the effective decontamination of environments exposed to radioactive materials. Radiation can linger in various forms, contaminating surfaces, air, and even water supplies. Therefore, understanding how to properly clean and decontaminate your surroundings is essential for minimizing exposure and protecting health.

Understanding Contamination

Radioactive contamination occurs when radioactive particles settle on surfaces or are absorbed by materials. These particles can be released during a nuclear explosion or from fallout. Contamination can be categorized into two types: external and internal. External contamination involves particles on the surface of the skin or clothing, while internal contamination occurs when radioactive materials are ingested or inhaled. The primary goal of decontamination is to remove these particles and reduce radiation exposure.

Basic Steps for Decontamination

1. Assess the Situation: Before beginning the decontamination process, assess the level of contamination. Use a radiation detector, if available, to identify contaminated areas. This will help prioritize which surfaces and objects require immediate attention.

2. Personal Protection: Prior to starting any decontamination efforts, ensure that you are wearing protective clothing. This includes gloves, masks, and goggles to minimize the risk of inhaling or coming into contact with radioactive particles.

3. Remove Contaminated Materials: Begin by safely removing items that are heavily contaminated and cannot be cleaned effectively. This may include clothing, textiles, and non-essential items. Place these items in securely sealed bags for disposal.

4. Wash Surfaces: For surfaces such as countertops, floors, and walls, use a combination of soap and water to scrub away contaminants. A solution of mild detergent can be effective. Work from the least contaminated areas toward more contaminated ones to avoid spreading radioactive particles.

5. Use a Wet Wipe Technique: For smaller objects, using damp cloths or disposable wipes can help trap radioactive particles. Wipe surfaces thoroughly and dispose of the wipes in sealed bags. Be sure to change wipes frequently to avoid recontamination.

6. Decontaminate Water Sources: If water sources are suspected to be contaminated, do not consume or use this water until it has been tested and deemed safe. Boiling water can kill pathogens, but it does not eliminate radioactive particles. Use filtration systems designed to remove contaminants or look for alternative clean water sources.

7. Ventilation: Increase airflow in indoor spaces to help dissipate any airborne radioactive particles. Open windows and doors to ventilate the area, but only if it is safe to do so without introducing additional contamination.

8. Monitor Radiation Levels: After decontaminating, continuously monitor radiation levels using detection devices. This ensures that the decontamination process was successful and identifies areas that may still require additional cleaning.

9. Long-Term Decontamination: For persistent contamination, consider applying more advanced techniques, such as using chemical decontaminants or seeking assistance from professionals if available. In severe cases, structural decontamination may be necessary, which could involve removing and replacing contaminated materials.

Conclusion
Decontaminating your environment after a nuclear event is essential for safety and health. By understanding the proper techniques and precautions, you can effectively reduce exposure to radioactive materials. It's crucial to maintain a vigilant approach, regularly assess contamination levels, and remain informed about best practices for decontamination. In a post-nuclear world, preparedness and knowledge are your best allies in ensuring safety and survival.

Chapter 9

Water and Food Safety in a Nuclear Environment

Identifying Contaminated Water Sources

In a post-nuclear environment, ensuring access to safe drinking water is paramount for survival. Contaminated water can lead to severe health issues, including gastrointestinal illnesses and long-term exposure to radioactive materials. Recognizing unsafe water sources and knowing how to respond is crucial for maintaining health and safety.

1. Recognizing Unsafe Water Sources:

Visual Indicators:
The first step in identifying contaminated water is to observe its physical characteristics. Unsafe water may appear cloudy or discolored, ranging from yellowish to brown. The presence of floating debris, sediment, or oily films on the surface can indicate contamination. If you notice an unusual smell, such as a chemical or rotten odor, it is a strong indication that the water is not safe to drink.

Location Considerations:
Understanding the source of the water is vital. Water from natural sources such as rivers, lakes, or ponds can be contaminated by runoff from surrounding areas, especially after a nuclear event. Areas near industrial sites, agricultural fields, or urban centers are more susceptible to chemical pollutants. Additionally, water collected from rooftops or other surfaces may be contaminated by fallout or debris.

Biological Indicators:
Even if water looks clear, it may still harbor harmful microorganisms. In a crisis, avoid water that is stagnant, as it is more likely to contain bacteria, parasites, and viruses. If you notice dead animals or excessive algae growth nearby, this can be another sign of contamination.

2. Testing for Contaminants:
When possible, use a water testing kit to evaluate water quality. These kits can detect chemical pollutants, bacterial contamination, and radiation levels. If you do not have access to a testing kit, consider the following improvised methods:

- **Smell and Taste Test:** Never ingest water that has an off-putting smell or taste, as this can indicate the presence of harmful substances.
- **Observation:** After pouring water into a clear container, let it sit for a few minutes. If sediment settles at the bottom, it may indicate contamination.

3. What to Do About Contaminated Water:

If you suspect that your water source is unsafe, it is critical to take immediate action:

- **Avoid Drinking:** Do not consume water that you suspect to be contaminated. Even small amounts can pose significant health risks.
- **Find Alternative Sources:** Look for other potential water sources, such as rainwater, which can be collected in clean containers. Ensure that collection surfaces are free from contamination.
- **Purification Methods:** If no clean water sources are available, use purification techniques to make the water safer for consumption. Boiling water for at least one minute (longer at higher altitudes) effectively kills most pathogens. Chemical treatments, such as chlorine tablets or iodine, can also be used, but make sure to follow the instructions carefully.

4. Long-Term Solutions:

In a post-nuclear environment, establishing a reliable water supply is paramount. Consider creating a water filtration system using sand, charcoal, and gravel to filter out impurities. Additionally, seek to build a rainwater harvesting system to collect and store clean water.

Conclusion:

Identifying contaminated water sources is a critical survival skill in a nuclear crisis. By recognizing unsafe water through visual, location, and biological indicators, employing testing methods, and knowing how to purify water, you can safeguard your health and increase your chances of survival. Prioritize finding and maintaining access to safe drinking water, as it is essential for sustaining life in any post-catastrophe scenario.

Purifying Water: Techniques and Tools

In the aftermath of a nuclear incident, access to clean water becomes paramount for survival. Water sources may be contaminated with radioactive materials, chemicals, or pathogens, making purification essential for health and safety. This section details various techniques and tools for making water safe to drink, ensuring that individuals and communities can secure this vital resource.

1. Boiling

Boiling is one of the simplest and most effective methods of purifying water. Heating water to a rolling boil for at least one minute (or three minutes at altitudes above 6,500 feet) kills most pathogens, including bacteria, viruses, and parasites. However, boiling does not remove chemical contaminants or heavy metals, which may require alternative purification methods.

Tools Needed:
- A heat source (camp stove, fire, or portable burner)
- A pot or container to hold water

Procedure:
1. Collect water in a clean container.
2. Heat the water until it reaches a rolling boil.
3. Maintain the boil for the recommended time.
4. Let the water cool before drinking or storing it in sanitized containers.

2. Filtration

Water filtration systems can effectively remove impurities and some contaminants. Portable water filters, such as those with activated carbon or ceramic elements, are widely available and can remove bacteria, protozoa, and some chemicals.

Tools Needed:
- Portable water filter (e.g., pump filter, gravity filter, or straw filter)
- Clean containers for collecting filtered water

Procedure:
1. Follow the manufacturer's instructions for the filter.
2. Pour or pump water through the filter into a clean container.
3. Ensure the filtered water is stored in a sanitary and sealed container to prevent recontamination.

3. Chemical Purification

Chemical treatments, such as chlorine or iodine tablets, can disinfect water effectively. These chemicals kill bacteria and viruses, making water safe to drink. However, they may not eliminate all parasites or chemical contaminants.

Tools Needed:
- Water purification tablets (chlorine or iodine)

- Clean containers for water

Procedure:
1. Fill a clean container with water.
2. Add the recommended number of purification tablets based on the water volume.
3. Stir the water and let it sit for the specified time (usually 30 minutes to 4 hours, depending on the chemical used).
4. Ensure the water is clear before consuming; if it smells too strong of chemicals, let it air out before drinking.

4. Solar Water Disinfection (SODIS)

SODIS is a sustainable method that utilizes sunlight to purify water. Clear, PET plastic bottles can be filled with contaminated water and left in direct sunlight for six hours (or up to two days in cloudy weather). UV rays from the sun kill pathogens.

Tools Needed:
- Clear PET plastic bottles
- Access to sunlight

Procedure:
1. Fill clean plastic bottles with water.
2. Place the bottles in direct sunlight, ensuring they are exposed to UV rays.
3. After the designated time, the water will be safer to drink.

5. Activated Carbon Filtration

Activated carbon can adsorb impurities and chemicals, improving water taste and odor. While it may not remove all pathogens, it can significantly enhance water quality.

Tools Needed:
- Activated carbon (available in granulated or powdered form)
- A filtration system or homemade filter setup (coffee filter, cloth, etc.)

Procedure:
1. Create a filter by layering activated carbon between cloth or coffee filters in a clean container.
2. Pour contaminated water through the filter.
3. Collect the filtered water in a separate container.

Conclusion

Water purification is a critical skill in a post-nuclear environment where access to clean water may be compromised. Using boiling, filtration, chemical treatments, solar disinfection, and activated carbon methods, individuals can make water safe to drink. It is crucial to assess the type of contamination present and choose the most appropriate purification method. By equipping oneself with knowledge and tools for water purification, survival and resilience in the face of adversity can be significantly enhanced.

Safe Food Sources: What to Eat and What to Avoid

In the aftermath of a nuclear explosion, the safety of food sources becomes a critical concern. Contamination from radioactive fallout can render many food items unsafe for consumption, posing serious health risks. Understanding what to eat and what to avoid is essential for survival in a post-nuclear environment. This section will guide you on how to identify safe food sources and the precautions necessary to ensure your diet remains as healthy as possible.

Understanding Contamination

Radioactive fallout can contaminate soil, water, and vegetation. The primary concern is that radioactive isotopes can be absorbed by plants and animals, entering the food chain. Foods grown in contaminated soil or exposed to contaminated water are at risk. Additionally, livestock that have ingested contaminated feed or water can carry radiation in their meat, milk, and eggs.

Identifying Safe Food Sources

1. Canned and Packaged Foods: In a post-nuclear scenario, canned and vacuum-sealed foods are among the safest choices. These items are sealed from the environment and have a long shelf life. Look for products stored in a safe area away from potential fallout. Ensure that canning materials are intact to avoid spoilage.

2. Root Vegetables: Root vegetables such as potatoes, carrots, and turnips can be safer options, provided they are grown in uncontaminated soil. If you have a garden, consider planting these crops in safe locations, avoiding areas where fallout might settle. Clean them thoroughly before consumption.

3. Wild Foraging: Foraging for wild edibles can be a viable source of nutrition, but caution is paramount. Avoid areas that could be contaminated. Focus on non-leafy plants (like berries and nuts) which are less likely to absorb radiation compared to leafy greens. Use a reliable guide to identify safe foraged foods and avoid any mushrooms, as they can absorb toxins from the soil.

4. Fish and Game: Catching fish or hunting game may be necessary for survival, but it is crucial to assess the risks. Fish from contaminated waters should be avoided. Game animals can also be carriers of radiation if they have ingested contaminated feed or water. If possible, test the meat for radiation levels before consumption.

5. Hydroponics and Indoor Gardening: If resources allow, consider setting up a hydroponic system or indoor garden. This method enables you to grow food in a controlled environment, minimizing exposure to contaminated soil and water. Use purified water to irrigate your plants and ensure they receive adequate light and nutrients.

Foods to Avoid

1. Leafy Greens: Vegetables like lettuce, spinach, and other leafy greens are at a higher risk of absorbing radiation directly from contaminated soil and water. It is advisable to avoid these until you can confirm the safety of the growing conditions.

2. Dairy Products: Milk and other dairy products from livestock that may have grazed on contaminated pastures should be avoided. Radiation can concentrate in the fat of animals, making dairy potentially hazardous.

3. Grains and Cereals: Unprocessed grains and cereals can also absorb toxins from the soil, making them unsafe. If you have access to grains, ensure they are sourced from uncontaminated areas.

4. Processed Foods: Foods that are heavily processed may contain ingredients from contaminated sources. Always check the origin of these products, and when in doubt, discard them.

Conclusion
In a contaminated environment following a nuclear event, careful selection of food sources is vital for survival. Prioritize canned goods, root vegetables, and foraged items from safe areas while avoiding potentially contaminated foods. Regularly assess your food sources for safety and stay informed about the levels of radiation in your environment. By taking these precautions, you can better ensure your health and well-being in a challenging post-nuclear landscape.

Growing Food Post-Nuclear Attack

In the aftermath of a nuclear attack, the landscape of survival shifts dramatically, particularly when it comes to securing food sources. One of the most pressing challenges is how to grow food in soil that may be contaminated with radioactive particles. Understanding how to cultivate crops safely and effectively in such conditions is vital for long-term survival.

Understanding Soil Contamination

Radioactive contamination in soil can occur through fallout, which consists of radioactive particles that settle on the ground after a nuclear explosion. These particles can remain hazardous for extended periods, making it critical to assess the level of contamination before attempting to grow food. Initial steps should include using a Geiger counter or similar radiation detection device to gauge radiation levels in the soil. Local authorities or community groups may also provide information about radiation levels in the area.

Soil Remediation Techniques

Before planting, it is essential to consider soil remediation techniques that can help reduce contamination levels. Some methods include:

1. Soil Removal: If the contamination is localized, physically removing the top layer of soil (the most contaminated) may be feasible. This is labor-intensive but can significantly reduce the risk of radiation exposure.

2. Phytoremediation: Certain plants, known as hyperaccumulators, can absorb heavy metals and some radioactive isotopes from contaminated soil. By planting these species, you can help extract harmful substances from the ground over time. Common hyperaccumulators include sunflowers and mustard plants.

3. Amending the Soil: Adding organic matter, such as compost or biochar, can help bind radioactive particles and reduce their bioavailability to plants. This not only improves soil health but may also decrease the concentration of contaminants that plants can uptake.

4. Building Raised Beds: Constructing raised garden beds filled with uncontaminated soil can create a safe planting environment. This method allows you to control the soil quality and reduce direct contact with contaminated ground.

Selecting Crops

Choosing the right crops is another critical aspect of growing food in contaminated soil. Opt for plants with low uptake of contaminants, particularly those that are less likely to absorb heavy metals and radioactive isotopes. Root vegetables, such as carrots and potatoes, tend to absorb more contaminants than leafy greens or fruits. Therefore, consider planting crops that are primarily above ground, such as:

- **Leafy Greens:** Lettuce, kale, and spinach can be suitable options, but they should be grown in raised beds with clean soil.
- **Fruits:** Crops such as tomatoes, peppers, and beans may also be beneficial, as their fruiting bodies are generally less prone to contamination than roots.

Additionally, you might consider planting perennial plants that can tolerate difficult conditions and provide food year after year, such as fruit trees or berry bushes.

Safe Harvesting Practices
When it comes time to harvest, employ safe practices to minimize exposure to any potential contaminants. Wear gloves and a mask to protect yourself from direct contact with soil or produce. After harvesting, wash all fruits and vegetables thoroughly with clean water to remove any surface contaminants. Cooking produce can also help reduce the risk of ingestion of harmful particles, as heat can kill many pathogens and help eliminate surface residues.

Community Collaboration
In a post-nuclear scenario, community collaboration becomes invaluable. Sharing knowledge about safe agricultural practices, distributing uncontaminated seeds, and pooling resources can enhance food security. Establishing community gardens or cooperative farming initiatives can also promote resilience and ensure that individuals have access to safe, nutritious food.

Conclusion
Growing food post-nuclear attack in contaminated soil is fraught with challenges, but through careful assessment, remediation techniques, crop selection, and safe harvesting practices, it is possible to cultivate food sources that are safe for consumption. By prioritizing community collaboration and collective knowledge, individuals can enhance their chances of survival and contribute to rebuilding a sustainable food system.

Storing and Preserving Food Safely
In the aftermath of a nuclear event, securing a reliable food supply is paramount for survival. The preservation and storage of food not only ensure sustenance but also minimize the risk of contamination from radiation and other environmental hazards. This section provides essential strategies for effectively storing and preserving food to maintain its safety and nutritional value.

1. Understanding Food Preservation Techniques

There are several methods for preserving food, each suited to different types of food and available resources. The most common methods include:

- **Canning:** This process involves sealing food in airtight containers and heating them to kill bacteria and enzymes that cause spoilage. It is vital to use proper canning techniques to prevent botulism, a potentially fatal illness caused by improperly canned foods.

- **Freezing:** Freezing food halts the growth of microorganisms and helps retain nutrients. However, in a post-nuclear scenario, reliable power sources may be scarce. Consider alternative freezing methods, such as buying dry ice or using solar-powered freezers, if available.

- **Dehydrating:** Removing moisture from food inhibits bacterial growth. Dehydration can be achieved through the use of a dehydrator, an oven set at low temperatures, or naturally through air drying in a sunny, dry environment.

- **Fermenting:** This method uses beneficial bacteria to convert sugars into acids, preserving food. Common fermented foods include sauerkraut, kimchi, and yogurt. Fermentation not only extends shelf life but also enhances nutritional value.

2. Choosing the Right Containers

Proper storage containers are crucial for maintaining food safety. The following types are recommended:

- **Glass Jars:** Ideal for canning and storing dry goods, glass jars are non-reactive and help keep out moisture and pests. Ensure they are properly sealed with lids designed for canning.

- **Food-Grade Plastic Containers:** Available in various sizes, these containers are useful for bulk storage of dry goods. Ensure they are BPA-free and airtight.

- **Mylar Bags:** For long-term storage, particularly for dehydrated or dry goods like rice and beans, Mylar bags with oxygen absorbers can prevent spoilage and pest infestation.

- **Coolers and Insulated Bags:** In the absence of electricity, insulated containers can help maintain colder temperatures for perishable items for a longer duration.

3. Creating a Safe Storage Environment

Food storage must be conducted in a clean, dry environment to prevent contamination. **Here are key steps to consider:**

- **Temperature Control:** Store food in a cool, dark place. Ideal temperatures range between 50°F and 70°F (10°C to 21°C). If possible, avoid areas that are prone to temperature fluctuations.

- **Humidity Control:** High humidity can promote mold and spoilage. Use desiccants or silica gel packets in storage areas to absorb excess moisture.

- **Pest Prevention:** Ensure that storage areas are sealed off from pests. Inspect food supplies regularly for signs of infestation, and use traps if necessary.

4. Labeling and Rotation

To maximize food safety and minimize waste, adopt a systematic approach to labeling and rotation:

- **Labeling:** Clearly label all containers with the contents and the date of storage. This practice helps track shelf life and ensures that older items are used first.

- **FIFO Method:** Implement the "First In, First Out" (FIFO) method. Consistently use older supplies before newer ones to ensure nothing goes to waste.

5. Monitoring Food Quality

Regularly assess the quality of stored food. Look for signs of spoilage, such as off-odors, discoloration, or changes in texture. In cases of doubt, it is better to err on the side of caution and dispose of questionable food.

By adopting these food storage and preservation strategies, individuals can significantly enhance their chances of sustaining themselves and their families in the challenging conditions following a nuclear event. Properly stored food not only provides essential nutrition but also contributes to mental well-being through the assurance of having adequate supplies during uncertain times.

Chapter 10

Communication and Information Gathering

Setting Up a Communication Network

In the unfortunate event of a nuclear conflict, maintaining communication becomes paramount for survival, coordination, and emotional support. A robust communication network enables individuals and communities to share critical information, plan collective responses, and sustain morale. Here, we will explore strategies for establishing and maintaining effective communication in a disrupted environment.

1. Establishing Communication Channels

a. Identify Available Technologies:
Before an incident occurs, familiarize yourself with various communication tools that can function in low-tech or disrupted environments. These may include:

- **Two-Way Radios:** Walkie-talkies or ham radios can provide short-range communication. Invest in a quality set that operates on multiple frequencies.
- **Satellite Phones:** These devices offer reliable connectivity even when traditional cell networks fail.
- **Emergency Flares or Signal Mirrors:** In dire situations, visual signals can be used to attract attention and communicate presence.

b. Create a Communication Plan:
Develop a clear plan that outlines how communication will occur among family members and friends. **This plan should include:**

- **Designated Meeting Points:** Agree on specific locations to regroup if separated.
- **Check-In Times:** Establish regular intervals for checking in with each other, whether through radio or other means.
- **Message Sending Protocols:** Create a system for sending messages, such as using code words or established phrases to convey specific information quickly and clearly.

2. Building a Community Network

a. Engage with Neighbors:
Communicate with those living nearby to establish a local network. Share contact information and discuss mutual interests in preparedness. This network can act as a support system during crises, allowing for resource sharing and collective problem-solving.

b. Form Communication Teams:
Encourage the formation of small groups within your community, each responsible for different aspects of communication. Some may focus on gathering information, while others may relay updates or coordinate supplies.

3. Utilizing Alternative Information Sources
In the aftermath of a nuclear incident, conventional news sources may be compromised. Therefore, diversifying information sources is crucial:

- **Local Radio Stations:** Tune into emergency broadcasts for updates from local authorities. A battery-operated radio can be invaluable.
- **Community Bulletin Boards:** Establish physical or digital boards where residents can post important messages, updates, and resource availability.
- **Word of Mouth:** Encourage community members to share updates with each other, especially in the absence of electronic devices.

4. Ensuring Reliability and Redundancy

a. Test Communication Equipment:
Regularly test radios, phones, and other devices to ensure they are operational. Practice using these devices so that everyone knows how to utilize them effectively in a crisis.

b. Backup Power Solutions:
In the event of power outages, have a backup power plan in place. Consider solar chargers for phones or radios, and stockpile batteries for devices that require them.

5. Training and Drills
Conduct regular training sessions and drills with your family and community to practice emergency communication protocols. This preparation will enhance familiarity with equipment and procedures, reducing panic and confusion during an actual event.

6. Handling Misinformation

During a crisis, misinformation can spread rapidly, exacerbating fear and confusion. Establish guidelines for verifying information before disseminating it. Encourage community members to rely on trusted sources and to report any conflicting information to a central authority within the network.

Conclusion

Establishing and maintaining a communication network in a disrupted environment requires foresight, planning, and collaboration. By leveraging technology, fostering community ties, and focusing on training and reliability, individuals can ensure that they remain connected and informed during times of crisis. This connectivity not only aids in survival but also enhances the collective resilience of communities facing the daunting challenges of a post-nuclear world.

Using Radios and Other Tools for Communication in a Post-Nuclear Environment

In the aftermath of a nuclear event, effective communication becomes crucial for survival. Not only does it provide a means to receive vital information, but it also helps maintain connections with loved ones and coordinate community efforts. In such scenarios, traditional communication infrastructure may be severely compromised, making alternative devices essential. This section explores various radios and other tools that can be used for both receiving and transmitting information in a post-nuclear environment.

1. Battery-Powered and Hand-Crank Radios

Battery-powered radios are indispensable in emergencies. These devices can pick up AM and FM signals and, importantly, NOAA weather channels that broadcast emergency information and weather updates. When selecting a radio, consider those that also feature a hand-crank option; this allows you to generate power manually if batteries run low. Some models come with additional features such as built-in flashlights and phone charging capabilities, thus serving multiple purposes in one device.

2. Two-Way Radios (Walkie-Talkies)

Two-way radios, commonly known as walkie-talkies, provide an excellent means of local communication without relying on external networks. They operate on radio frequencies and are particularly useful for short-range communication among groups. When selecting two-way radios, prioritize models with a long battery life and a variety of channels to minimize interference. In a community setting, establishing a set of designated channels for different groups can enhance coordination and situational awareness.

3. Amateur (Ham) Radios

Ham radios are a more advanced communication tool, requiring a license to operate. However, they offer significant advantages during crises. These radios can transmit over long distances, allowing communication with other operators far from the immediate area. They can also tap into emergency services and established networks that may still be operational post-disaster. Joining local amateur radio clubs before a crisis can provide valuable training and build relationships with experienced operators, enhancing your preparedness.

4. Satellite Phones

In a situation where terrestrial networks are down, satellite phones can be lifelines. They connect directly to satellites rather than cell towers, allowing communication even in remote areas. While they are more expensive and may require subscriptions, their ability to function independent of local infrastructure makes them invaluable during a nuclear aftermath. Acquiring one ahead of time and familiarizing yourself with its use can be a significant advantage.

5. Communication Apps and Devices

If the internet remains operational, various communication apps on smartphones can facilitate messaging and voice calls. Tools like WhatsApp, Signal, or even email can be used to communicate quickly and efficiently. Note that these tools rely on battery power and internet access, making them less reliable than radios in a complete blackout scenario. However, having portable solar chargers can extend the usability of such devices significantly.

6. Emergency Beacons and Personal Locator Beacons (PLBs)

Emergency beacons are crucial for sending distress signals. PLBs can transmit GPS coordinates to search and rescue teams, making them an essential tool for those venturing outside their immediate shelter. These devices are compact and battery-operated, and they can be lifesavers if you find yourself in a situation where you cannot communicate by other means.

Conclusion

In a post-nuclear environment, having a range of communication tools at your disposal is vital for survival. Investing in battery-powered radios, two-way radios, ham radios, satellite phones, and emergency beacons can significantly improve your ability to receive vital information and connect with others. Preparing these tools ahead of time, along with understanding their operation, can enhance resilience and foster community cooperation in the face of adversity. Communication is not just about exchanging information; it is a lifeline that can aid in recovery and rebuilding efforts in a profoundly altered world.

Establishing Contact with Authorities

In the chaotic aftermath of a nuclear event, establishing contact with authorities becomes essential for survival and recovery. The ability to receive accurate information, access resources, and report critical situations can significantly influence your safety and that of your loved ones. Here, we will explore various methods for reaching out to government sources and how to effectively gather information during such a crisis.

Understanding the Communication Landscape

In the aftermath of a nuclear explosion, traditional communication channels may be disrupted. This can include the failure of phone lines, internet outages, and the unavailability of radio broadcasts. Understanding the landscape of communication methods available to you is the first step toward establishing contact with authorities.

1. Emergency Broadcast Systems: Many regions have emergency broadcast systems designed to disseminate critical information during disasters. Familiarize yourself with local emergency frequencies and how to access them. Battery-operated or hand-crank radios can be invaluable for receiving updates in the absence of electricity.

2. Mobile Networks: While mobile phone networks may be congested or damaged, text messaging often remains a viable option. Text messages require less bandwidth than voice calls and may go through when traditional calls do not. Keep your messages brief and to the point to conserve space on the network.

3. Community Communication Networks: Establishing a network within your community can provide a reliable source of information. Neighbors can share updates, and local leaders may have more immediate access to information from government sources. Create a plan for regular check-ins or information exchanges to keep everyone informed.

Reaching Out to Authorities

When re-establishing contact with governmental bodies, consider the following strategies:

1. Local Emergency Services: Identify local emergency services, including police, fire departments, and emergency management agencies. These organizations often have designated channels for public communication. Look for official announcements on social media platforms or community bulletin boards.

2. Government Hotlines: Many governments provide hotlines during disasters for citizens to report emergencies or seek assistance. Familiarize yourself with these numbers beforehand, ensuring you have them saved in a secure and accessible location.

3. Official Websites and Social Media: In a post-nuclear environment, official government websites and social media accounts can be crucial for real-time updates. When the internet is available, check these sources for announcements, safety instructions, and resource availability.

4. Community Meetings: Attend community meetings organized by local authorities or civic groups. These gatherings can be platforms for sharing critical information, resources, and safety protocols. They also provide an opportunity to voice concerns and ask for assistance.

Verifying Information

In the aftermath of a nuclear event, misinformation can spread rapidly. Therefore, verifying the information you receive is crucial:

1. Cross-Reference Sources: Before acting on any information, cross-reference it with multiple credible sources. If possible, compare updates from government agencies with community reports to ascertain their accuracy.

2. Listen to Official Messages: Pay close attention to information conveyed through official channels. Government announcements regarding safety protocols, evacuation procedures, and medical assistance will be crucial for your immediate well-being.

3. Community Feedback: Engage with your community to validate information. If several individuals have heard similar messages from different sources, it may indicate a higher likelihood of accuracy.

Conclusion

Establishing contact with authorities in the wake of a nuclear event is a multifaceted process that requires preparation, adaptability, and vigilance. By understanding available communication methods, proactively reaching out to government sources, and verifying information, you can ensure that you and your community stay informed and safe in the critical moments that follow. In such uncertain times, the ability to communicate effectively with authorities can make a significant difference in navigating the challenges of survival and recovery.

Finding Reliable Information: Avoiding Misinformation

In the chaotic aftermath of a nuclear event, the ability to access accurate and reliable information becomes paramount for survival. Misinformation can spread rapidly, exacerbating panic and leading to poor decision-making during critical times. This section will explore strategies to identify trustworthy sources, verify information, and ensure that you are equipped with the most accurate data available.

1. Identifying Trusted Sources

The first step in finding reliable information is to recognize which sources are credible. Trusted sources typically include:

- **Government Agencies:** National and local emergency management agencies (such as FEMA in the United States) provide official updates and guidelines during crises. Their information is often vetted and reliable.
- **Established News Organizations:** Reputable news outlets with a history of journalistic integrity can be valuable. Look for organizations that are known for their fact-checking protocols and ethical standards.
- **Non-Governmental Organizations (NGOs):** Reputable NGOs, especially those focused on humanitarian aid and disaster response, can provide accurate information and resources.
- **Experts and Professionals:** Academics, scientists, and professionals in relevant fields (e.g., emergency management, public health) often share valuable insights. Look for expert opinions published in peer-reviewed journals or recognized platforms.

2. Verifying Information

Once you have identified potential sources, verifying the information is crucial. **Here are steps to ensure accuracy:**

- **Cross-Reference Information:** Check multiple sources to see if the information is consistent. If several trusted outlets report the same facts, it's more likely to be accurate.
- **Check the Date:** In emergencies, outdated information can lead to dangerous decisions. Always verify the publication date of the information to ensure its relevance.
- **Look for Citations:** Credible information often cites original research, studies, or official statistics. If a source makes claims without backing them up, approach it with skepticism.
- **Be Aware of Bias:** Every source may have its biases, especially in emotionally charged situations. Evaluate whether the information presented is balanced or if it seems to promote a specific agenda.

3. Using Technology Wisely
In a post-nuclear scenario, technology can be both a tool and a trap:

- **Social Media Vigilance:** While social media platforms can provide real-time updates, they are also notorious for spreading misinformation. Be cautious and verify claims before sharing or acting on them.
- **Reliable Apps and Websites:** Utilize apps designed for emergency management, which provide alerts and updates from credible sources. Websites like the CDC, WHO, or specific government emergency management sites are often reliable.
- **Emergency Broadcast Systems:** In many countries, emergency alert systems can provide crucial information during crises. These systems are generally reliable—pay attention to them for updates.

4. Engaging with the Community
Post-attack, fostering community connections can enhance information reliability:

- **Community Meetings:** Participate in local gatherings or discussions to share information and updates. A community-based approach can help in filtering out misinformation and reinforcing shared knowledge.
- **Local Networks:** Establish communication networks with neighbors or community groups. They can serve as a resource for verifying information and sharing updates.

5. Maintaining Critical Thinking
Above all, maintaining a mindset of critical thinking is essential:

- **Question Everything:** Always ask yourself who is providing the information, why they might be sharing it, and how they might be influenced by their own biases or interests.
- **Stay Calm:** Panic can cloud judgment and lead to hasty decisions based on unreliable information. Take a moment to evaluate the situation and the information at hand before acting.

In conclusion, navigating the landscape of information during a nuclear crisis demands vigilance, skepticism, and community engagement. By identifying trusted sources, verifying information, using technology wisely, and maintaining critical thinking, individuals can significantly enhance their ability to make informed decisions in the face of uncertainty.

The Role of Community Networks

In the aftermath of a nuclear event, individuals and families will face unprecedented challenges that can overwhelm even the most prepared survivalist. However, the strength of community networks can be a powerful lifeline during these critical times. Building and relying on local networks for survival and information is not only vital for physical sustenance but also essential for emotional resilience and social cohesion. This section explores how to establish these networks, the benefits they offer, and strategies for mobilizing community resources effectively.

Establishing Community Networks

1. Identify Local Resources and Skills: Begin by mapping out the skills and resources within your community. This includes identifying individuals with expertise in various survival skills such as gardening, first aid, construction, and security. Hosting community meetings can facilitate introductions and allow members to share their skills and resources. Creating a directory of contact information can streamline communication.

2. Create Communication Channels: In the event of a nuclear crisis, traditional means of communication may be disrupted. Establishing alternative communication channels, such as neighborhood radios, message boards, or local bulletin boards, can help keep everyone informed. Forming small groups or committees dedicated to information dissemination can enhance clarity and reduce misinformation.

3. Regular Training and Drills: Hosting regular survival training sessions and emergency drills can strengthen community bonds while ensuring everyone is prepared. These activities foster trust and cooperation, allowing community members to practice skills such as first aid, fire safety, and emergency preparedness.

4. Form Alliances with Local Organizations: Leverage existing community organizations, such as neighborhood associations, faith groups, and local nonprofits, to build a broader network. These organizations often have established communication channels and resources that can be mobilized in times of crisis.

The Benefits of Community Networks

1. Resource Sharing: In a post-nuclear environment, resources such as food, water, and medical supplies will be scarce. Community networks enable the pooling of resources, allowing members to share what they have and access a wider array of supplies. This collective approach can significantly enhance survival prospects.

2. Emotional Support: The psychological toll of a nuclear event can be devastating. Community networks provide a support system where individuals can share their fears, grief, and anxieties. Group gatherings and discussions can foster understanding and help individuals cope with the emotional fallout of such a crisis.

3. Collective Security: A united community can better protect itself from external threats. Establishing watch groups or patrols can enhance safety and deter potential dangers. A cohesive network allows for greater vigilance, creating a sense of security among members.

4. Information Dissemination: In a crisis, timely and accurate information is crucial. Community networks can facilitate the rapid spread of important updates regarding safety, resource availability, and any potential threats. This can help prevent panic and misinformation from spreading.

Strategies for Mobilizing Community Resources

1. Organize Regular Meetings: Schedule regular gatherings to discuss community needs, share updates, and develop strategies for mutual aid. These meetings can serve as both planning sessions and social gatherings, reinforcing community ties.

2. Implement a Buddy System: Pair community members with one another to ensure no one is left isolated. Buddies can check on each other's well-being, share resources, and provide emotional support.

3. Develop a Community Emergency Plan: Collaborate to create a comprehensive emergency plan that outlines how the community will respond to various scenarios, including resource distribution, sheltering, and communication strategies. This plan should be revisited and updated regularly.

4. Encourage Inclusivity: Ensure that all community members feel welcome and valued in the planning process. Diverse perspectives can enhance problem-solving and create a stronger, more resilient network.

In conclusion, community networks play an indispensable role in survival and recovery following a nuclear event. By fostering connections, sharing resources, and offering mutual support, communities can not only endure the immediate challenges but also lay the groundwork for rebuilding a sustainable future. Together, individuals can create a resilient framework that transforms a crisis into an opportunity for collaboration, hope, and healing.

Chapter 11

Psychological Resilience and Mental Health

Coping with Isolation and Loneliness

In the aftermath of a nuclear conflict, the psychological impacts of isolation and loneliness can be profound. These feelings can arise from the loss of community, loved ones, and the familiar structures of daily life. Understanding and proactively addressing these challenges is essential for maintaining mental health during such trying times. Here are several strategies to cope with isolation and loneliness effectively.

1. Establish a Routine

Creating a daily routine provides structure and a sense of normalcy amidst chaos. A routine can include basic tasks such as meal preparation, hygiene, exercise, and leisure activities. By establishing a schedule, individuals can create a semblance of control over their environment, which can reduce feelings of uncertainty and anxiety. Even simple actions like making your bed, planning meal times, or setting aside specific times for reading or hobbies can foster a sense of accomplishment and purpose.

2. Engage in Creative Expression

Creative outlets can be powerful tools for coping with isolation. Engaging in activities such as drawing, writing, music, or crafting can help individuals express their emotions and process their experiences. Journaling, for example, can serve as a means to articulate thoughts and feelings, providing an emotional release and facilitating self-reflection. Likewise, creative projects can distract from loneliness, allowing for moments of joy and fulfillment even in difficult circumstances.

3. Cultivate Mindfulness and Meditation

Mindfulness practices can significantly benefit mental health by promoting present-moment awareness and reducing anxiety about the future. Techniques such as deep breathing, meditation, and yoga can help calm the mind and improve emotional regulation. Setting aside time each day for mindfulness exercises can foster a sense of peace and help individuals reconnect with themselves, mitigating feelings of loneliness and despair.

4. Maintain Connections

While physical distancing may be necessary, maintaining emotional connections is crucial. Utilize available communication tools such as radios, satellite phones, or other means to stay in touch with loved ones and community members. Establishing a routine for checking in with others can provide mutual support and foster a sense of belonging. Whether through conversations, shared activities, or even collaborative projects, maintaining these connections can significantly alleviate feelings of isolation.

5. Develop a Support Network

Building a local support network can create a sense of community and shared purpose. Engage with neighbors or other survivors to form small groups where individuals can share resources, skills, and emotional support. Group activities, such as communal meals or collective planning, can foster a sense of solidarity and help combat loneliness. Establishing trust and open communication within this network can be instrumental in navigating the challenges of post-nuclear life.

6. Focus on Physical Health

Physical well-being is closely linked to mental health. Engage in regular physical activities, whether through structured exercise or simply walking outside when safe. Maintaining a balanced diet can also enhance mood and energy levels. Prioritizing sleep and rest is crucial, as fatigue can exacerbate feelings of loneliness and depression. Taking care of the body can provide a strong foundation for mental resilience.

7. Seek Professional Help When Possible

If access to mental health professionals is available, seeking support from trained individuals can be invaluable. Therapy or counseling can provide strategies to cope with trauma, loss, and feelings of loneliness in a safe environment. If formal help is inaccessible, consider reaching out to trusted friends or community members who can offer emotional support.

In conclusion, coping with isolation and loneliness in a post-nuclear world requires proactive strategies that foster mental resilience. By establishing routines, engaging in creative expression, maintaining connections, and prioritizing physical health, individuals can navigate the psychological challenges of isolation, ultimately promoting mental well-being even in the most challenging circumstances.

Managing Stress and Anxiety Post-Attack

In the aftermath of a nuclear attack, the psychological repercussions can be as devastating as the physical destruction. Managing stress and anxiety becomes paramount for survival and recovery. The chaotic and uncertain environment following such an event can lead to heightened anxiety levels, making it essential to adopt effective coping strategies. This section outlines several practical techniques to help individuals manage ongoing stress and anxiety in a post-attack scenario.

1. Establish a Routine

Creating a structured daily routine can provide a sense of normalcy amidst chaos. Routines help individuals regain a sense of control over their lives, which is crucial for mental well-being. Incorporate regular activities such as meal preparation, exercise, and scheduled communication with family members. Even simple tasks like morning hygiene or setting times for rest can provide essential stability.

2. Practice Mindfulness and Relaxation Techniques

Mindfulness practices, such as meditation and deep-breathing exercises, can significantly reduce stress and anxiety. These techniques focus on grounding oneself in the present moment, helping to alleviate feelings of fear and worry about the future. Spend a few minutes each day practicing deep, slow breaths, or engage in mindfulness meditation by concentrating on your breath or surrounding sounds. Apps or guides can support these practices, even in a resource-scarce environment.

3. Engage in Physical Activity

Physical activity is a powerful stress reliever. In a post-attack scenario, find ways to incorporate exercise into daily life. This could be through simple exercises like stretching, walking, or improvised workouts using available resources. Physical movement releases endorphins, which can elevate mood and reduce feelings of anxiety. It also helps maintain physical health, which is vital in a recovery situation.

4. Maintain Social Connections

Isolation can exacerbate feelings of anxiety and depression. Maintaining connections with family, friends, and community members is essential. Create a communication plan to check in regularly with loved ones. Engage in discussions about feelings and experiences, as sharing can help normalize emotions and provide mutual support. If community structures are still functional, participating in group activities can foster a sense of belonging and collective resilience.

5. Limit Exposure to Stressors

While it's important to stay informed, constant exposure to distressing news can heighten anxiety. Set boundaries around media consumption, whether through radio, newspapers, or conversations. Allocate specific times for checking updates and avoid continuous exposure to potentially triggering information. This can help manage the emotional impact of ongoing threats.

6. Focus on Problem-Solving

In the face of uncertainty, it can be beneficial to shift focus from overwhelming feelings of anxiety to actionable problem-solving. Identify immediate challenges and prioritize addressing them, whether it's securing food, ensuring water safety, or establishing shelter. By taking proactive steps, individuals can feel more empowered and less helpless, which can significantly reduce anxiety levels.

7. Seek Professional Help, If Possible

In cases where anxiety and stress become overwhelming, seeking professional help can be invaluable. While access to mental health services may be limited post-attack, connecting with trained individuals through community organizations or emergency services can offer critical support. Crisis hotlines or local support groups, if available, can provide guidance and reassurance.

8. Cultivate Hope and Positivity

Lastly, fostering a mindset of hope is vital. Focus on small victories and progress made in recovery. Engage in activities that bring joy or comfort, whether through creative pursuits, storytelling, or shared meals. Maintaining a positive outlook can serve as a powerful antidote to the pervasive anxiety that may arise in the aftermath of a nuclear attack.

By implementing these techniques, individuals can create a foundation for managing stress and anxiety effectively, enhancing their ability to cope with the challenges of a post-nuclear world.

Dealing with Grief and Loss

In the aftermath of a nuclear event, the emotional landscape can be as devastating as the physical destruction. The loss of loved ones and the obliteration of familiar life can lead to profound grief, making it essential to develop effective coping strategies. Understanding grief and its manifestations can aid individuals in navigating this challenging emotional terrain.

Understanding Grief

Grief is a natural and complex emotional response to loss, encompassing a range of feelings such as sadness, anger, confusion, and despair. In the immediate aftermath of a nuclear event, individuals may experience shock and disbelief, which can numb the pain temporarily. However, as reality sets in, the depth of loss becomes apparent, leading to a cycle of emotional highs and lows. It's crucial to recognize that grief is not linear; it unfolds uniquely for each person, influenced by their relationship with the deceased, personal coping mechanisms, and the surrounding environment.

Acknowledging the Pain
One of the first steps in coping with grief is to acknowledge the pain. Suppressing emotions can lead to prolonged suffering and manifest in various physical and psychological issues. Encourage self-reflection and allow yourself to feel the full spectrum of emotions, from sorrow to anger. Journaling can be a helpful tool, providing an outlet for expressing feelings and processing thoughts about the loss. Writing down memories of loved ones can also serve as a tribute, preserving their legacy and fostering a sense of connection amidst the chaos.

Seeking Support
In times of grief, social connections become even more critical. While the instinct may be to isolate oneself, reaching out to others who have shared the experience can foster healing. Forming support groups with fellow survivors can create a space for shared stories, allowing individuals to express their feelings, validate each other's experiences, and offer mutual support. If community networks are disrupted, consider leveraging technology to connect with friends or family outside the immediate situation, as remote communication can provide a lifeline.

Establishing New Routines
The loss of loved ones often disrupts daily life, creating a void that can feel insurmountable. Establishing new routines can provide a sense of normalcy and purpose. Engage in activities that promote physical health, such as exercise or gardening, which can also serve as therapeutic outlets. Setting small, achievable goals can help instill a sense of accomplishment and gradually rebuild confidence and resilience in the face of overwhelming grief.

Honoring Their Memory
Finding ways to honor the memory of lost loved ones can be a powerful coping mechanism. Creating rituals, such as lighting a candle, planting a tree, or celebrating their birthdays with small remembrances, can provide comfort and a tangible connection to the past. Engaging in acts of kindness or community service in their honor can also transform grief into positive action, fostering a sense of purpose and connection to others.

Professional Help
While community support can be invaluable, professional help may be necessary for some individuals. Mental health professionals can provide coping strategies tailored to individual needs and help navigate complex grief reactions. In a post-nuclear world, where resources may

be scarce, seeking out teletherapy or community mental health initiatives can bridge the gap in access to care.

Conclusion
Coping with grief in a post-nuclear world is a profound journey that requires patience, understanding, and support. By acknowledging pain, seeking connection, establishing new routines, honoring memories, and utilizing professional resources when needed, individuals can begin to navigate their grief. While the loss of loved ones and the life once known may feel overwhelming, fostering resilience and community can pave the way for healing in a drastically altered world.

Maintaining Hope: Finding Purpose and Meaning
In the aftermath of a nuclear conflict, the landscape of daily life can be irrevocably altered, leaving individuals in a state of despair, uncertainty, and emotional turmoil. Maintaining hope and finding purpose in such dire circumstances is not only essential for psychological resilience but also for fostering community cohesion and rebuilding society. Here, we explore practical strategies to cultivate hope and meaning during these challenging times.

Understanding the Importance of Hope
Hope serves as a crucial psychological buffer against the overwhelming stress and trauma that follows catastrophic events. It can facilitate recovery, inspire action, and cultivate a sense of agency in individuals and communities. Psychologists emphasize that hope is a dynamic process that involves setting goals, developing pathways to achieve those goals, and maintaining motivation despite obstacles. In a post-nuclear world, this process becomes vital as individuals strive to reclaim their lives and rebuild their communities.

Setting Realistic Goals
One of the first steps in fostering hope is to set achievable, short-term goals. These goals can range from immediate survival tasks—such as securing food and water—to longer-term objectives like establishing a community garden or rebuilding essential infrastructure. By focusing on small, manageable tasks, individuals can experience a sense of accomplishment that reinforces their belief in their ability to effect change. Setting realistic goals also encourages cooperation and collaboration, as community members can work together towards common objectives, fostering social bonds and shared purpose.

Engaging in Meaningful Activities
Engaging in activities that provide a sense of purpose can significantly enhance motivation and hope. This might include volunteering to help others in the community, participating in

rebuilding efforts, or creating art and literature that reflects the experiences and emotions of those affected by the nuclear event. Such activities not only provide a distraction from trauma but also help individuals process their experiences and promote healing. Creating spaces for community gatherings and sharing stories can further reinforce social ties and instill a sense of belonging.

Cultivating Resilience through Adaptation

Resilience—the ability to adapt to adversity—can be cultivated through practice and mindset shifts. Encouraging a focus on flexibility and adaptability can help individuals navigate the uncertainties of a post-nuclear world. This might involve learning new skills, such as foraging, gardening, or self-defense, which can empower individuals and enhance self-sufficiency. By embracing the idea that adaptation is possible, individuals can find strength in the belief that they can overcome challenges, leading to a renewed sense of hope.

The Role of Community

Community support plays a critical role in maintaining hope and purpose. Building networks of support enables individuals to share resources, knowledge, and emotional support. Communities can organize regular meetings to discuss challenges and brainstorm solutions, fostering a collective sense of agency. Peer support groups can also be instrumental in providing a safe space for individuals to express their feelings, fears, and aspirations. The act of coming together not only alleviates feelings of isolation but also reinforces the notion that individuals are not alone in their struggles.

Spirituality and Personal Reflection

For many, spirituality can provide a profound source of hope and meaning during the darkest times. Engaging in spiritual practices—be they prayer, meditation, or reflection on personal values—can help individuals find solace and strength. Personal reflection on past experiences and the lessons learned can also foster a sense of purpose and guide future actions. By contemplating what is truly important in life, individuals can reorient their focus towards rebuilding and healing.

Conclusion

In a world reshaped by a nuclear event, maintaining hope and finding purpose is paramount. By setting realistic goals, engaging in meaningful activities, cultivating resilience through adaptation, fostering community connections, and embracing spirituality, individuals can navigate the complexities of their new reality. Hope is not merely a passive feeling but an active pursuit that can inspire individuals to rebuild their lives and communities, creating a foundation for a brighter future.

The Importance of Community and Support Systems

In the aftermath of a nuclear event, the world as we know it can become profoundly altered, leading to heightened anxiety, uncertainty, and fear. In such dire circumstances, the importance of community and support systems cannot be overstated. These networks play a crucial role in fostering mental and emotional resilience, enabling individuals and families to navigate the complexities of survival and recovery effectively.

The Role of Community

Communities serve as the foundation for collective resilience. In a post-nuclear scenario, the shared experiences, skills, and resources of community members become vital. A strong community can provide not only physical support—like shared food and water supplies—but also emotional backing, which is essential for mental health. Being part of a group helps individuals feel less isolated, as they can share their fears and experiences, ultimately leading to a sense of belonging and purpose.

Building Support Networks

To build effective support networks, individuals should take proactive steps before a crisis occurs. This involves identifying neighbors, friends, and local organizations that can provide assistance and companionship. Here are several strategies for establishing robust community connections:

1. Engage in Community Activities: Participate in local events, meetings, and volunteer opportunities. This engagement builds relationships and fosters trust among community members.

2. Create Communication Channels: Establish reliable means of communication, such as group chats, community bulletin boards, or ham radio networks. These channels can facilitate quick information sharing during emergencies.

3. Organize Skills Workshops: Hosting workshops can help community members learn essential survival skills, such as first aid, food preservation, and self-defense. Sharing knowledge not only empowers individuals but strengthens community bonds.

4. Form Support Groups: Establishing support groups for mental and emotional health can provide a safe space for individuals to express their feelings and concerns. Facilitated discussions can help people cope with trauma and stress collectively.

5. Develop Emergency Plans Together: Collaboratively creating emergency plans that outline roles, resources, and communication strategies can enhance preparedness and build confidence within the community.

Relying on Support Systems

Once support networks are established, individuals must recognize the value of relying on these systems during crises. Support systems can help mitigate feelings of helplessness and despair by providing:

- **Emotional Support:** Sharing experiences and feelings with others can alleviate the psychological burden often associated with traumatic events. Listening and validating each other's feelings fosters an environment of understanding and compassion.

- **Practical Assistance:** Community members can pool resources, such as food, water, and medical supplies, ensuring that no one is left to fend for themselves. This collective approach can enhance the overall survival rate.

- **Shared Knowledge and Skills:** By leveraging the diverse skills present within a community, individuals can learn from one another, ensuring that everyone is equipped to face the challenges ahead. This diversity can also spark innovation in problem-solving.

- **A Sense of Normalcy:** In a chaotic environment, the presence of a supportive community can help restore a sense of normalcy. Regular gatherings or meetings can provide structure and routine, which are crucial for mental stability.

Conclusion

In the face of unprecedented challenges posed by a nuclear event, the importance of community and support systems emerges as a beacon of hope. By actively building and nurturing these networks, individuals can cultivate a resilient environment that not only supports survival but also promotes healing and growth. Together, communities can transform fear into strength, fostering a collective spirit that emphasizes compassion, cooperation, and the relentless pursuit of a better future. In rebuilding after catastrophe, it is the bonds forged in adversity that will ultimately guide society toward resilience and renewal.

Chapter 12

Rebuilding Society Post-Nuclear War

The Challenges of Rebuilding: Where to Start

In the aftermath of a nuclear war, the enormity of the challenges faced by survivors can be overwhelming. The immediate devastation, characterized by widespread destruction, loss of life, and psychological trauma, creates a daunting environment for rebuilding. Identifying key priorities is essential for effective recovery and to foster resilience in affected communities. Here, we will outline several critical areas that need urgent attention and action.

1. Assessing Immediate Needs and Safety

The first step in rebuilding is to ensure the safety and survival of those who remain. This involves conducting a thorough assessment of the immediate environment for hazards, including radiation levels, structural damage, and potential hazards from debris. Establishing safe zones for survivors, where radiation levels are manageable and basic needs can be met, is paramount. Access to clean water, food, and medical care must be prioritized to prevent further loss of life and to stabilize the community.

2. Restoration of Basic Services

Once immediate safety is established, the focus shifts to restoring essential services. This includes re-establishing water and sanitation systems, electricity, and communication networks. In many cases, local infrastructure will be damaged or entirely destroyed, necessitating innovative solutions and potential external aid. Temporary solutions, such as portable water purification systems and solar-powered generators, may provide the necessary stopgap measures until permanent infrastructure can be rebuilt.

3. Health Care and Psychological Support

The health care system will likely be strained or non-existent in the wake of a nuclear disaster. Addressing both physical injuries and the psychological impact of the event is crucial. Survivors may experience acute radiation sickness, injuries from the blast, and significant mental health challenges stemming from trauma and loss. Establishing makeshift clinics and ensuring access to medical supplies, as well as mental health support systems, must be a priority. Community-based approaches, such as support groups and counseling services, can significantly aid in the healing process.

4. Food Security and Agriculture

Food shortages are likely to occur after a nuclear event due to disrupted supply chains and agricultural damage. Prioritizing food security involves assessing local resources and implementing immediate measures for food distribution. Long-term strategies might include community gardens, sustainable farming techniques, and foraging education to ensure that communities can produce their own food. This not only addresses hunger but also fosters community collaboration and resilience.

5. Establishing Governance and Law

The breakdown of traditional governance structures can lead to chaos and lawlessness. Re-establishing some form of governance is critical for maintaining order and providing a framework for decision-making. This could involve forming community councils that include diverse voices, ensuring representation and fairness. Clear communication about laws and expectations can help mitigate conflicts and establish a sense of normalcy.

6. Rebuilding Community and Social Structures

Social cohesion is vital for recovery. The trauma experienced by survivors can create divisions if not addressed properly. Initiatives to rebuild community ties through collaborative projects, shared resources, and communal activities can help restore a sense of belonging and purpose. Encouraging open dialogues about experiences and losses can foster healing and solidarity among community members.

7. Learning from the Past

Finally, it is essential to reflect on lessons learned from historical case studies of nuclear events, such as Hiroshima and Nagasaki. Understanding past recovery efforts can provide valuable insights into effective rebuilding strategies and potential pitfalls to avoid. This historical perspective can also inform future preparedness plans to ensure communities are better equipped to handle similar crises.

In conclusion, rebuilding after a nuclear war requires a multifaceted approach that prioritizes safety, health, food security, governance, and community resilience. By addressing these key areas, survivors can begin the arduous journey toward recovery, ultimately fostering a stronger and more united society in the face of adversity.

Infrastructure Recovery: Power, Water, and Transportation

In the aftermath of a nuclear war, the restoration of critical infrastructure is paramount for survival, stability, and the gradual rebuilding of society. The three essential components—power, water, and transportation—serve as the backbone of recovery efforts. Each of these elements is deeply interconnected; without reliable electricity, clean water becomes difficult to purify and distribute, while transportation systems are essential for moving resources and people.

Power Restoration

The first step in restoring power is assessing the damage to the electrical grid. Nuclear explosions can cause widespread destruction to power plants and transmission lines, leading to significant outages. Communities must prioritize the restoration of local energy sources, beginning with smaller, decentralized systems such as solar panels, wind turbines, and generators powered by alternative fuels. While large-scale power plants may take time to rehabilitate, microgrids can provide an immediate solution, enabling localized energy production and distribution.

Communities should form collaboration networks to pool resources, knowledge, and skills. Skilled tradespeople—electricians, engineers, and technicians—must be mobilized to repair damaged infrastructure. Government agencies or local authorities can facilitate these efforts by providing resources, information, and support for the workforce.

Additionally, it is crucial to implement energy conservation measures to reduce demand during the initial recovery phase. Encouraging residents to limit energy use, along with the adoption of energy-efficient appliances, can help ensure that the available power is sufficient for critical needs, such as medical facilities and food storage.

Water Recovery

Access to clean water is one of the most pressing concerns following a nuclear event. Contamination from radioactive fallout can render existing water sources unsafe, necessitating the establishment of new systems for water procurement, purification, and distribution. Communities should first assess existing water supplies, including groundwater and surface water sources, to determine their safety for consumption.

Methods for purifying water must be prioritized. Boiling water is one of the simplest and most effective ways to eliminate pathogens, while other techniques include filtration and chemical treatment. Communities can utilize portable water purification systems and encourage the use of rainwater harvesting systems to supplement water supplies.

In the long term, rebuilding the water infrastructure will require collaboration with engineers and water management experts to design and implement systems that are both resilient and sustainable. This may involve the creation of new treatment plants or the rehabilitation of existing facilities to ensure safe drinking water.

Transportation Recovery

Transportation infrastructure is critical for facilitating the movement of goods, people, and aid. Roads, bridges, and railways may have suffered extensive damage due to explosions and subsequent fallout. An immediate assessment of transportation routes is necessary to identify which can be repaired and which may require complete reconstruction.

Communities should prioritize the restoration of key transportation links to facilitate the flow of essential supplies, including food, medical supplies, and equipment needed for recovery efforts. Establishing clear communication channels to coordinate transportation efforts is vital, as is the formation of volunteer groups that can assist in debris removal and road repairs.

In addition to reopening existing channels, communities might consider innovative solutions like bicycle networks or pedestrian pathways to ensure mobility while larger-scale transportation systems are restored. This can help reduce reliance on fuel and promote community engagement.

Conclusion

The recovery of critical infrastructure—power, water, and transportation—requires a coordinated effort involving local communities, skilled professionals, and government support. By prioritizing immediate needs and fostering resilience through decentralized solutions, societies can lay the groundwork for long-term recovery and stability. In the face of adversity, these foundational elements will be vital for nurturing life and rebuilding hope in a post-nuclear world.

Establishing Governance and Law

In the aftermath of a nuclear war, the immediate challenges of survival are often compounded by the breakdown of established political and social structures. Rebuilding governance and law is crucial to restoring order, ensuring the protection of individual rights, and facilitating cooperation among survivors. This section outlines the steps necessary for establishing effective governance in a post-nuclear society.

Assessing the Situation

The first step in rebuilding governance is to assess the current situation. This involves understanding the extent of destruction, the availability of resources, and the needs of the populace. Engaging with local communities to gather insights into their immediate concerns and aspirations is essential. This participatory approach not only fosters trust but also ensures that the governance structures established are reflective of the community's needs.

Forming a Leadership Structure

While formal government bodies may no longer exist, local leaders often emerge naturally in times of crisis. These leaders can be anyone from community elders to former officials who possess the experience and respect of the populace. Establishing a council or committee, composed of diverse representatives from various sectors of the community, can facilitate more inclusive decision-making. It is crucial to ensure that this leadership structure embodies transparency and accountability to gain the community's trust.

Creating a Legal Framework

Once a leadership structure is in place, the next step is to establish a legal framework to govern behavior and resolve conflicts. This framework should prioritize fundamental human rights and community safety. Drawing upon pre-existing laws and adapting them to the new realities can provide a starting point. Additionally, community-based conflict resolution mechanisms, such as mediation and restorative justice practices, can be effective in fostering cooperation and social cohesion.

Restoring Order and Security

One of the immediate challenges in a post-nuclear environment is maintaining order and security. This can be achieved through the establishment of local law enforcement groups that are trained to protect rather than oppress. Community policing efforts, where local citizens participate in safety initiatives, can help maintain order while fostering trust between the populace and those in power.

Moreover, clear communication about laws and expectations is essential. This includes disseminating information about rights, responsibilities, and the processes for reporting crimes or grievances. Utilizing community meetings, flyers, and communication networks can help ensure that everyone is informed.

Encouraging Civic Participation

Rebuilding governance is not solely the responsibility of leaders; civic participation is vital. Encouraging community members to take an active role in decision-making processes can enhance the legitimacy of governance structures. This can be achieved through regular town hall meetings, public forums, and participatory budgeting initiatives. Such practices empower individuals, foster a sense of ownership, and cultivate a culture of responsibility and cooperation.

Establishing Alliances and Cooperation

In a post-nuclear context, the rebuilding of governance must also extend beyond local communities to foster regional alliances and cooperation. Establishing networks with neighboring communities can help share resources, knowledge, and support. These alliances can also work towards creating regional governance structures that are more resilient and better equipped to handle larger-scale challenges.

Long-Term Vision and Adaptability

Finally, it is crucial to adopt a long-term vision for governance that is adaptable to changing circumstances. The governance structures and laws established in the immediate aftermath may need to evolve as conditions improve and societal needs change. Continuous evaluation and adaptation of these systems will ensure that they remain relevant and effective.

In conclusion, rebuilding governance and law in a post-nuclear society is a multifaceted process that requires community engagement, clear legal frameworks, security measures, and long-term adaptability. By prioritizing inclusivity and cooperation, communities can develop resilient governance structures that protect individual rights, maintain order, and foster a sense of collective responsibility essential for survival and recovery in a challenging new world.

Restoring Education and Healthcare

In the aftermath of a nuclear catastrophe, the restoration of essential social services, particularly education and healthcare, is pivotal in rebuilding a stable and functioning society. Both sectors are fundamental to ensuring community resilience, fostering social cohesion, and promoting overall well-being amidst the challenges of a post-nuclear world.

Healthcare Restoration

The healthcare system will face unprecedented challenges following a nuclear event. Immediate injuries from radiation exposure, burns, and trauma will strain medical resources. Hospitals and clinics may be damaged or destroyed, necessitating the establishment of temporary medical facilities and mobile clinics to provide urgent care. The first priority must be to train laypersons in basic first aid and triage methods, enabling them to manage injuries while professional healthcare workers are mobilized.

Healthcare professionals must focus on managing radiation sickness, where symptoms can vary from nausea and vomiting to severe fatigue and skin burns. Establishing protocols for treating both acute and long-term health effects of radiation exposure is crucial. This includes monitoring for delayed effects such as cancers and other diseases associated with radiation. To facilitate treatment, communities should prioritize the stockpiling of essential medical supplies, including antibiotics, pain relievers, and radiation treatment drugs, ensuring their availability for those in need.

Mental health is another critical aspect of post-nuclear recovery. The trauma experienced during and after a nuclear event can lead to widespread psychological issues, including PTSD, anxiety, and depression. Community-based mental health support systems should be established, focusing on peer support, counseling, and coping strategies. Training community leaders and volunteers to recognize mental health issues and provide support can significantly enhance resilience within the population.

Education Restoration

Education is not only essential for the intellectual development of children but also for fostering critical thinking, problem-solving, and social skills necessary for rebuilding society. The immediate aftermath of a nuclear event will disrupt conventional schooling, necessitating alternative educational approaches.

Community centers can be transformed into makeshift schools, offering basic education to children and adults alike. Curriculum should focus on practical skills relevant to survival, such as agriculture, healthcare basics, and trade skills, preparing the populace for the realities they will face in a resource-scarce environment. Emphasizing science education, particularly in areas related to health and safety, can empower individuals to make informed decisions about their well-being in a contaminated world.

In addition, fostering a culture of lifelong learning through community workshops and skills training can help rebuild the social fabric. Engaging community members in teaching their skills can create a sense of ownership and responsibility toward collective recovery. As the community begins to stabilize, formal educational institutions can gradually be restored, integrating traditional subjects with practical life skills to prepare future generations for a world altered by nuclear events.

Collaboration and Resource Sharing

The successful restoration of healthcare and education will require collaboration among various stakeholders, including local governments, non-governmental organizations (NGOs), and international aid agencies. Sharing resources, expertise, and best practices will be vital in creating a robust framework for recovery.

Establishing partnerships with organizations experienced in disaster recovery can facilitate the provision of necessary materials and expertise. Furthermore, engaging local and regional leaders in the decision-making process ensures that the restored services align with the community's needs and cultural values.

In conclusion, the restoration of education and healthcare in a post-nuclear society is a complex but essential endeavor. By prioritizing immediate health needs, focusing on mental well-being, and creating adaptable educational frameworks, communities can rebuild not just their infrastructure but also their spirits, fostering resilience and hope for the future.

The Role of International Aid and Cooperation

In the aftermath of a nuclear catastrophe, the immediate and long-term recovery of affected regions hinges significantly on international aid and cooperation. The scale of devastation caused by a nuclear event is unparalleled, often resulting in not only physical destruction but also profound psychological and social impacts. In such circumstances, the collaborative efforts of nations, international organizations, non-governmental organizations (NGOs), and local communities become critical to restoring stability and initiating recovery processes.

Immediate Humanitarian Assistance

In the wake of a nuclear disaster, the priority is to address the urgent humanitarian needs of survivors. International aid can provide essential resources such as food, water, medical supplies, and shelter. Organizations like the United Nations and the International Red Cross have established frameworks for rapid response in emergencies, enabling them to mobilize resources and deploy medical and logistical teams swiftly. These organizations work in tandem with local governments and NGOs to assess needs, distribute supplies, and provide medical care to those affected by radiation exposure and injuries.

Infrastructure Rehabilitation

The destruction of infrastructure, including hospitals, schools, and transportation systems, presents a formidable challenge in post-nuclear recovery. International cooperation is vital for rebuilding these essential services. Countries with the capacity to offer technical expertise and financial support can assist in reconstructing critical infrastructure. This can involve the sharing of advanced engineering practices, rebuilding techniques that prioritize safety against future radiation hazards, and ensuring that new facilities are equipped to handle disasters more effectively. Additionally, international financial institutions can provide loans and grants to support reconstruction efforts without overburdening the local economy.

Knowledge and Technology Transfer

One of the critical aspects of recovery involves the transfer of knowledge and technology. Countries that have experienced nuclear incidents, such as Japan after Fukushima, possess valuable insights into managing nuclear fallout, radiation health effects, and long-term environmental remediation. International collaboration allows for the sharing of best practices, research, and innovations in radiation safety, environmental monitoring, and public health strategies. This exchange of knowledge helps affected nations develop tailored recovery plans that are informed by both local and global experiences.

Mental Health and Psychological Support

The psychological toll of a nuclear disaster can be profound, with survivors facing trauma, anxiety, and grief. International aid can extend beyond physical reconstruction to include mental health support and counseling. Global mental health organizations can train local professionals to provide trauma-informed care, facilitate community healing programs, and create support networks for affected individuals. By fostering a sense of community and resilience, these initiatives can significantly enhance the recovery process.

Long-Term Development and Prevention

The role of international cooperation must also extend to long-term development strategies that address the root causes of vulnerability to nuclear disasters. Collaborative efforts can include the promotion of peace-building initiatives, disarmament discussions, and diplomatic efforts to prevent future nuclear conflicts. By engaging in dialogue and fostering trust among nations, the international community can work toward reducing the likelihood of nuclear warfare and enhancing global security.

Building a Culture of Preparedness

Finally, international aid and cooperation can foster a culture of preparedness, encouraging nations to invest in disaster preparedness and response strategies. Through joint training exercises, simulation drills, and the sharing of resources, countries can strengthen their ability to respond to potential nuclear threats. This proactive approach not only aids in immediate recovery but also builds resilience against future disasters, ensuring that societies are better equipped to handle crises.

In conclusion, the role of international aid and cooperation in the aftermath of a nuclear event is multifaceted and essential. Through humanitarian assistance, infrastructure rehabilitation, knowledge sharing, mental health support, long-term development, and preparedness strategies, global collaboration can significantly enhance recovery efforts, ultimately leading to a more resilient and unified global community in the face of potential nuclear challenges.

Chapter 13

Self-Defense and Security

Protecting Yourself and Your Family

In the grim reality of a post-nuclear world, the preservation of life extends beyond mere survival techniques; it encompasses ensuring the safety and security of oneself and loved ones against potential threats that may arise in the aftermath of a disaster. Understanding basic self-defense techniques and strategies is crucial, as the environment may become unpredictable, and societal norms could deteriorate, leading to increased hostility and competition for resources.

Awareness and Prevention

The first line of defense in any dangerous situation is awareness. Being vigilant and aware of your surroundings can help you identify potential threats before they escalate. This means tuning into the behaviors of others, recognizing the signs of aggression, and understanding the environment you inhabit. Developing a habit of situational awareness allows you to anticipate danger and react accordingly, giving you an advantage in avoiding confrontation whenever possible.

Verbal De-escalation Techniques

Before resorting to physical self-defense, employing verbal de-escalation techniques can be a powerful tool. Calmly addressing an aggressor with a non-confrontational demeanor may defuse tension. Use a steady voice and maintain eye contact, expressing empathy while firmly stating your position. Phrases like, "I understand you're upset, but let's talk this through calmly," can help shift the focus from confrontation to resolution. The goal is to diffuse hostility without escalating the situation further.

Physical Self-Defense Techniques

If a physical confrontation becomes unavoidable, understanding some basic self-defense techniques can empower you to protect yourself and your family effectively. Here are a few fundamental moves to consider:

1. Stance and Posture: Adopt a balanced and stable stance, with your feet shoulder-width apart. Keep your hands up in a defensive posture, ready to protect your face and body.

2. Targeting Vulnerable Areas: In a self-defense situation, aim for vulnerable areas of the attacker, including the eyes, nose, throat, and groin. Striking these areas can incapacitate an aggressor, providing you with a chance to escape.

3. Simple Strikes: Practice basic strikes such as palm strikes, elbow strikes, and knee strikes. These techniques utilize the body's natural weaponry and require minimal training.

4. Escape Techniques: Learn how to break free from holds or grips. Techniques such as twisting your body to escape a wrist grab or using leverage to disengage can be crucial.

5. Using Your Surroundings: In a survival scenario, everyday objects can become improvised weapons. Items such as keys, pens, or even a backpack can be used to create distance or defend yourself if necessary.

Family Safety Plans

Creating a comprehensive family safety plan is critical for ensuring the protection of loved ones. This plan should include designated meeting points, communication strategies, and emergency contacts. Role-playing scenarios with your family can help everyone understand their roles in various situations, fostering a sense of preparedness.

Building a Community Defense Network

In a post-nuclear world, fostering relationships with neighbors and creating a community defense network can enhance safety. Establishing a group of trusted individuals can provide mutual protection and support. Regular meetings to discuss safety concerns, share resources, and develop collective strategies can strengthen community ties and enhance security.

Ethical Considerations

While self-defense is essential, it's crucial to maintain a moral compass even in dire situations. Understanding the difference between self-defense and aggression is vital. The goal is to protect oneself and loved ones without resorting to unnecessary violence. Ethical considerations should guide your actions, ensuring that you remain humane even when faced with potential threats.

In conclusion, protecting yourself and your family in a post-nuclear scenario requires a combination of awareness, communication, and practical self-defense skills. By preparing mentally and physically for potential threats, you can enhance your ability to navigate a dangerous environment while prioritizing the safety of those you care about.

Securing Your Shelter Against Threats

In the aftermath of a nuclear event, securing your shelter becomes paramount to ensure the safety and survival of you and your loved ones. The threats you may face can range from radiation exposure to looters and other hostile individuals in a post-apocalyptic environment. Therefore, fortifying your living space is a critical step in preparation for both immediate and long-term survival.

1. Assessing Vulnerabilities

The first step in securing your shelter is to conduct a thorough assessment of its vulnerabilities. This includes examining doors, windows, vents, and any other points of entry. Identify weak spots where an intruder might gain access or where radiation could infiltrate. Consider the structural integrity of your shelter; if possible, opt for a basement or an underground bunker, as these locations naturally provide more protection from radiation and external threats.

2. Reinforcing Doors and Windows

Reinforcing doors and windows is essential for maintaining the security of your shelter. Solid-core doors are preferred over hollow-core doors, as they provide better resistance to forced entry. Install deadbolts and security bars to make it significantly harder for intruders to gain access. For windows, consider using security film or storm shutters to prevent shattering. Additionally, covering windows with heavy blankets or tarps can offer added protection against radiation and prying eyes, while also helping to insulate the shelter.

3. Creating Barriers

Building barriers can be an effective way to deter intruders and create a more secure environment. Consider constructing reinforced barricades using furniture, heavy items, or even makeshift barriers with materials like sandbags. These can be placed in front of entry points to slow down or stop any potential threats. If your shelter has a perimeter, enhance it with fencing or natural obstructions, such as thorny bushes, to discourage unwanted visitors.

4. Sealing Against Radiation

To protect against radiation, it is crucial to seal all potential entry points. Use weather stripping, caulk, or adhesive sealants to close gaps around doors, windows, and vents. Consider creating a decontamination area at the entrance of your shelter, where anyone entering can remove contaminated clothing and leave outside items behind to minimize the risk of bringing radiation indoors. This area should also have a method for cleaning footwear to prevent tracking in contaminants.

5. Establishing a Communication and Alarm System

In a post-nuclear scenario, communication can be a lifeline. Establish a reliable communication system within your shelter, using two-way radios or walkie-talkies to maintain contact with other members of your group. Additionally, set up an alarm system that can alert you to any unauthorized access. This could be a simple tripwire connected to bells or more advanced systems involving motion detectors.

6. Developing Self-Defense Strategies

Lastly, consider incorporating self-defense strategies into your overall security plan. Train yourself and your family members in basic self-defense techniques to prepare for potential encounters with threats. Having a self-defense tool, such as pepper spray or a baton, can provide an added layer of protection. Furthermore, understanding how to de-escalate a situation can be invaluable in avoiding confrontation.

Conclusion

Securing your shelter against potential threats in a post-nuclear world involves a multi-faceted approach that combines physical fortifications, strategic planning, and mental preparedness. By assessing vulnerabilities, reinforcing entry points, creating barriers, sealing against radiation, establishing communication systems, and developing self-defense strategies, you can create a secure environment that enhances your chances of survival. Preparation and vigilance are key; by taking these proactive steps, you can significantly improve your safety and resilience in the face of adversity.

Handling Unwanted Encounters

In a post-nuclear world, the social fabric may be frayed, leading to increased tensions and potential confrontations. Understanding how to handle unwanted encounters with hostile individuals is essential for survival and safety. This section will explore techniques for de-escalation and self-defense, emphasizing the crucial balance between maintaining personal safety and avoiding unnecessary conflict.

Understanding the Context

First, it is important to recognize the context in which these encounters may occur. After a nuclear event, resources such as food, water, and shelter will be in short supply. This scarcity can lead to heightened stress levels, desperation, and aggression among individuals. Being aware of this environment allows for a more informed approach to potential confrontations.

De-escalation Techniques

1. Remain Calm and Composed: The first rule of de-escalation is to maintain your composure. When faced with hostility, a calm demeanor can help diffuse tension. Take deep breaths, speak slowly, and use a steady tone. Your body language should be open and non-threatening; avoid crossing your arms or making sudden movements that could be perceived as aggressive.

2. Active Listening: Acknowledging the other person's feelings can significantly reduce hostility. Use active listening techniques—such as nodding, maintaining eye contact, and paraphrasing their concerns—to show that you are engaged and empathetic. This can help the other person feel heard and understood, which may lower their defensive posture.

3. Use "I" Statements: When addressing the situation, use "I" statements to express your feelings without sounding accusatory. For example, saying "I feel uncomfortable when you raise your voice" is less confrontational than "You are being aggressive." This approach can help shift the focus from blame to personal feelings, promoting understanding.

4. Establish Boundaries: If the situation continues to escalate despite your de-escalation efforts, calmly state your boundaries. Phrases like "I am not comfortable with this conversation" or "I need to walk away now" can assert your needs without exacerbating the aggression. Be clear but polite, as this can help maintain a level of respect.

5. Offer Alternatives: If possible, suggest alternative solutions to the conflict. Proposing a compromise or a different course of action can redirect the conversation and diffuse tension. For instance, if a person is demanding resources, you might suggest sharing what you can rather than engaging in a confrontation.

Self-Defense Techniques

In the unfortunate event that de-escalation fails and a confrontation turns physical, having self-defense techniques can be vital. While the goal is to avoid violence, it is important to be prepared.

1. Situational Awareness: Being aware of your surroundings can help you avoid potential threats before they escalate. Pay attention to body language and environmental cues that may indicate hostility. If something feels off, trust your instincts and remove yourself from the situation if possible.

2. Defensive Posture: If confronted, adopt a defensive posture. Keep your hands up, palms facing forward, to signal that you do not wish to engage in violence. This stance can convey readiness without appearing overly aggressive.

3. Target Vulnerable Areas: If physical confrontation is unavoidable, aim for vulnerable areas of the attacker, such as the eyes, throat, or groin. Striking these areas can incapacitate an aggressor and provide you with an opportunity to escape.

4. Escape First: The primary goal of self-defense should always be to escape the situation safely. Use any opportunity to flee rather than engage further. Look for exits and be aware of potential escape routes.

5. Seek Help: After a confrontation, report the incident to authorities or community leaders as soon as you can. Ensuring that hostile behavior is addressed can help maintain safety in your community.

In conclusion, the ability to manage unwanted encounters with hostile individuals through effective de-escalation and self-defense techniques is essential in a post-nuclear society. By prioritizing calm communication and understanding while being prepared to protect oneself, individuals can navigate these challenging situations with greater confidence and safety.

Building a Community Defense Network

In the wake of a nuclear conflict, the need for safety and security becomes paramount. One of the most effective strategies for ensuring protection is to establish a Community Defense Network (CDN). This network not only enhances safety through collective action but also fosters resilience among community members. Here are steps and considerations for organizing and participating in such a network.

Assessing Community Needs and Resources

The first step in building a CDN is to assess the specific needs and resources of your community. This can involve:

1. Mapping Community Assets: Identify individuals with skills relevant to survival and defense—medical professionals, security experts, educators, and those with experience in leadership or crisis management.

2. Understanding Vulnerabilities: Analyze the community's vulnerabilities, including potential threats from both external and internal sources. This might include assessing geographical risks, available infrastructure, and the socio-economic dynamics that could influence security.

3. Establishing Communication Channels: Create reliable communication methods to disseminate information quickly. This can include setting up a community bulletin board, a group messaging app, or regular community meetings. Ensuring that all members know how to communicate effectively is vital for coordinated efforts.

Formulating a Defense Strategy

Once the community's needs and resources are assessed, it's time to develop a defense strategy. This strategy should be comprehensive and adaptable:

1. Establishing Guidelines: Create a set of guidelines that outline the roles and responsibilities of community members during a crisis. This could include who to contact in emergencies, how to respond to potential threats, and procedures for evacuating vulnerable individuals.

2. Training and Drills: Organize training sessions where community members can learn essential skills such as first aid, self-defense, and emergency response techniques. Regular drills can help solidify these skills and ensure that everyone knows their role during an actual event.

3. Emergency Plans: Develop a clear plan for various scenarios, including natural disasters, social unrest, or nuclear fallout. This plan should include evacuation routes, designated safe zones, and points of contact for reporting emergencies.

Building Trust and Relationships

A successful CDN relies on trust and collaboration among its members. To foster this environment:

1. Encourage Participation: Invite community members to participate in discussions about security and defense. This inclusivity fosters a sense of ownership and responsibility towards the community's safety.

2. Facilitate Social Bonds: Organize social events that bring community members together. Building relationships in non-crisis times strengthens the fabric of the community and creates a support network when challenges arise.

3. Transparent Communication: Maintain open lines of communication about the community's defense strategies, successes, and challenges. Transparency builds trust and allows for collective problem-solving.

Engaging with External Resources
While the primary focus is on community resources, external support can significantly enhance a CDN:

1. Local Authorities and Organizations: Establish connections with local law enforcement, emergency services, and non-governmental organizations (NGOs) that can provide expertise, resources, or support during a crisis.

2. Training from Experts: Consider inviting experts in emergency preparedness and community defense to conduct workshops or training sessions. Their knowledge can offer invaluable insights and enhance the skills of community members.

3. Networking with Other Communities: Form alliances with neighboring communities to share resources, information, and strategies. This can provide a broader safety net and enhance the overall resilience of the region.

Conclusion
Building a Community Defense Network is not merely a reactive measure; it is a proactive approach to fostering resilience and security in uncertain times. By assessing community needs, formulating a comprehensive defense strategy, building trust, and engaging with external resources, communities can empower themselves to face the challenges that may arise in a post-nuclear world. Collaboration and preparation are essential, not just for survival, but for thriving together in the face of adversity.

Ethical Considerations in Self-Defense
In the aftermath of a nuclear war, survival instincts are likely to dominate human behavior. However, as individuals and communities navigate this new reality, it is crucial to consider the ethical implications surrounding self-defense. This section explores the delicate balance between ensuring personal safety and adhering to moral principles in a post-nuclear world.

The Right to Self-Defense
At its core, the concept of self-defense is rooted in the fundamental right to preserve one's life and well-being. In a post-apocalyptic scenario, where law and order may be compromised, the instinct to protect oneself and loved ones can drive individuals to take drastic measures.

However, the ethical justification of such actions often depends on the context and the means employed in self-defense.

Individuals must recognize that their actions may have significant consequences, not just for themselves but for their communities. The ethics of self-defense can be framed within the principles of necessity and proportionality. Actions taken in self-defense should be necessary to prevent imminent harm, and the degree of force used should not exceed what is reasonable to avert that threat. This balance is critical in maintaining moral integrity amid chaos.

Contextualizing Threats

In a post-nuclear world, threats may arise not only from external aggressors but also from desperate individuals or groups competing for limited resources. Understanding the motivations behind such threats can help inform ethical decision-making. For instance, an individual who approaches out of desperation rather than malice may not warrant the same response as someone exhibiting clear intent to harm.

The ethical approach to self-defense involves assessing the nature of the threat. Engaging in a dialogue to de-escalate a situation can be an ethical alternative to violence. Non-lethal measures should be prioritized whenever possible, as they can defuse tensions without resorting to fatal options. This approach not only upholds ethical standards but also contributes to a more stable community in the long term.

The Role of Community and Collective Defense

In the context of survival, the role of community becomes paramount. Ethical considerations in self-defense extend beyond individual actions to the collective responsibility of protecting vulnerable members of society. In a post-nuclear environment, individuals may need to form alliances and community defense networks to ensure mutual safety. This communal approach fosters a sense of shared responsibility and can mitigate the isolation that often accompanies survival scenarios.

Community defense strategies should emphasize cooperation and inclusivity. Establishing clear ethical guidelines for collective self-defense can help prevent abuses of power and promote accountability. Such guidelines could include protocols for conflict resolution, the equitable distribution of resources, and the protection of non-combatants.

Navigating Moral Dilemmas

The post-nuclear landscape will inevitably present a myriad of moral dilemmas, particularly regarding the use of force. Decisions made in the heat of the moment can lead to irreversible consequences. Individuals must cultivate moral readiness by reflecting on their values and the principles guiding their actions. Engaging in discussions about ethics within community groups can prepare individuals to face difficult decisions with a clearer moral compass.

Educating oneself about the implications of self-defense, including the potential for harm to others and the psychological toll it may take, is vital. Understanding the legal and ethical frameworks that govern self-defense can also inform personal actions and promote a culture of responsibility.

Conclusion

Ultimately, the ethical considerations surrounding self-defense in a post-nuclear world compel individuals to strike a balance between the instinct to survive and the moral duty to uphold humanity. By prioritizing non-violent solutions, engaging with communities, and preparing for moral dilemmas, individuals can navigate the challenges of survival with integrity and compassion. This commitment to ethical self-defense not only protects personal interests but also fosters a resilient society capable of rebuilding in the aftermath of catastrophe.

Chapter 14

Medical Care in a Post-Nuclear World

Managing Common Injuries: First Aid Essentials

In a post-nuclear war scenario, access to modern medical facilities may be severely limited or entirely unavailable. Therefore, knowledge of basic first aid is crucial for ensuring survival in a world where injuries and illnesses can arise from various sources, including radiation exposure, environmental hazards, and common accidents. This section outlines essential first aid techniques that can help individuals manage common injuries and illnesses without the benefit of modern healthcare.

Understanding Basic First Aid Principles

First aid refers to the immediate care provided to someone suffering from an injury or illness until professional medical help is available. The primary goals of first aid are to preserve life, prevent the condition from worsening, and promote recovery. Anyone can learn first aid techniques, and it is advisable to keep a well-stocked first aid kit handy, even in a post-apocalyptic setting.

Common Injuries and Their Management

1. Cuts and Scrapes:

   - Assessment: Determine the severity of the wound. If it's deep and bleeding profusely, apply direct pressure using a clean cloth or bandage.
   - Cleaning: Rinse the wound gently with clean water to remove dirt and debris. Avoid using alcohol or hydrogen peroxide initially as they can damage tissue.
   - Dressing: Cover the wound with a sterile bandage or cloth to prevent infection. Change the dressing regularly and monitor for signs of infection, such as redness, swelling, or pus.

2. Burns:

   - First-Degree Burns: For mild burns (redness and minor swelling), cool the area with running water for at least 10 minutes. Avoid ice, as it can further damage the skin. Apply aloe vera gel or a clean, non-stick dressing.

- **Second-Degree Burns:** For blisters and more severe burns, do not pop the blisters. Keep the area clean, cover it with a sterile dressing, and monitor for infection. Seek medical help if available.
- **Third-Degree Burns:** Do not attempt to treat severe burns with remedies. Cover the area with a clean cloth and seek professional help immediately.

3. Fractures and Sprains:
- **Fractures:** Immobilize the injured area with a makeshift splint using sturdy materials (e.g., sticks, rolled-up newspapers). Elevate the limb if possible and apply ice wrapped in cloth to reduce swelling. Avoid moving the person unless necessary.
- **Sprains:** Follow the R.I.C.E. method—Rest, Ice, Compression (with a bandage), and Elevation. Avoid putting weight on the injured joint.

4. Bleeding:
- **Minor Bleeding:** Apply direct pressure on the wound with a clean cloth. Elevate the area above the heart if possible.
- **Severe Bleeding:** If bleeding does not stop after 10 minutes of direct pressure, apply a tourniquet above the injury. Use only as a last resort and seek help immediately.

5. Infections:
- **Signs:** Fever, increased pain, swelling, and discharge can indicate infection.
- **Management:** Keep wounds clean and dry. Use herbal remedies such as honey or garlic, known for their antibacterial properties, if antibiotics are unavailable.

6. Dehydration and Heat Exhaustion:
- **Signs:** Symptoms include dizziness, dry mouth, and fatigue.
- **Management:** Encourage the affected person to rest in a cool area and sip small amounts of clean water or electrolyte-rich fluids. If severe, seek shade and apply cool cloths.

Mental Preparedness
In addition to physical treatment, it is essential to maintain a calm demeanor when providing first aid. Panic can exacerbate any situation, making it harder to think clearly. Encourage those around you to remain focused and collective in their efforts to assist those injured.

Conclusion
Mastering basic first aid skills is vital for survival in a post-nuclear world where medical resources may be scarce. By knowing how to treat common injuries and illnesses, individuals can increase their chances of recovery and contribute to the well-being of their communities.

Regular practice and familiarity with these skills can empower individuals and provide a sense of control in an unpredictable environment.

Treating Radiation Sickness and Burns

Radiation sickness, also known as acute radiation syndrome (ARS), occurs when a person is exposed to a high dose of ionizing radiation, typically from a nuclear explosion, accident, or medical treatment. The severity of radiation sickness depends on the dose received and the duration of exposure. Understanding the symptoms and appropriate treatment methods is critical for survival in a post-nuclear environment.

Recognizing Radiation Sickness

Symptoms of radiation sickness can manifest within hours or days following exposure. Early signs include:

1. Nausea and Vomiting: These are often the first symptoms to appear. They may start within minutes to hours after exposure and can persist for days.
2. Diarrhea: This symptom can occur in conjunction with nausea and vomiting, leading to dehydration.
3. Fatigue and Weakness: Affected individuals may feel unusually tired or weak, which can worsen over time.
4. Skin Burns: Depending on the intensity of exposure, radiation can cause skin burns that may appear red and blistered.
5. Hair Loss: High doses of radiation can lead to hair loss within weeks of exposure.
6. Neurological Symptoms: In severe cases, individuals may experience confusion, disorientation, or loss of consciousness.

Immediate Management of Radiation Sickness

If radiation sickness is suspected, it is essential to take immediate action:

1. Decontamination: Remove contaminated clothing and wash the skin thoroughly with soap and water to remove radioactive particles. This can help reduce the risk of further radiation exposure.
2. Hydration: Encourage the affected person to drink plenty of fluids to combat dehydration, especially if they are experiencing nausea and diarrhea.
3. Symptomatic Relief: Anti-nausea medications, if available, can help alleviate vomiting. Over-the-counter pain relievers may also assist with headaches or body aches.
4. Rest: Ensure the affected person rests in a safe, quiet environment to aid recovery and reduce stress.

Treating Radiation Burns

Radiation burns can vary in severity and require specific care:

1. Mild Burns (First-Degree): These burns can be treated with cool compresses and aloe vera or other soothing lotions. Over-the-counter pain relievers can help manage discomfort.

2. Moderate Burns (Second-Degree): For blisters or deeper tissue damage, it's important to avoid breaking blisters, as this can lead to infection. Cover the area with sterile, non-adhesive dressings and seek medical attention when possible.

3. Severe Burns (Third-Degree): If the burn is extensive or involves deeper layers of skin, immediate medical care is necessary. In a post-nuclear environment, prioritize infection prevention by keeping the area clean and covered.

Long-Term Management Considerations

The effects of radiation exposure may not be immediately apparent. Long-term monitoring for symptoms of radiation-induced illnesses is crucial. These may include:

- **Increased Cancer Risk:** Individuals exposed to significant radiation may face a higher risk of developing certain cancers, necessitating regular medical check-ups.
- **Chronic Health Issues:** Long-term effects can include cardiovascular problems, cataracts, and other health complications related to radiation exposure.

Conclusion

Recognizing and managing the symptoms of radiation sickness and burns is vital in the aftermath of a nuclear event. Immediate decontamination, hydration, and symptomatic relief can significantly improve outcomes for affected individuals. As the situation stabilizes, ongoing care and monitoring for long-term health impacts will be necessary to ensure survival and recovery. Understanding these principles can empower individuals and communities to respond effectively in the face of a nuclear threat.

Dealing with Chronic Conditions without Modern Medicine

In the aftermath of a nuclear event, the disruption of healthcare systems poses a significant challenge for individuals managing chronic conditions. With limited access to modern medicine, it becomes crucial to adapt and develop strategies to maintain health and manage symptoms effectively. Here are key considerations and strategies for coping with chronic illnesses in a resource-scarce environment.

Understanding Your Condition

The first step in managing chronic conditions without modern medicine is to have a comprehensive understanding of your illness. This includes knowing the symptoms, triggers, and potential complications associated with your condition. Keeping a detailed record of your health history, including previous treatments and their effectiveness, can provide valuable insights that may guide your self-care practices in a crisis.

Creating a Personalized Management Plan

Develop a personalized health management plan tailored to your condition. This plan should include:

1. Symptom Recognition: Be vigilant about recognizing early signs of flare-ups or complications. This awareness allows for timely interventions to prevent worsening conditions.

2. Lifestyle Adjustments: Identify lifestyle changes that can mitigate symptoms. For example, if you have diabetes, focus on maintaining stable blood sugar levels through diet and exercise, even when resources are limited.

3. Alternative Therapies: Explore alternative therapies that may help alleviate symptoms. Practices such as meditation, yoga, and herbal remedies may provide relief and improve overall well-being. However, it is essential to research these options to ensure they are safe and appropriate for your condition.

Resource Management

In a resource-scarce environment, managing supplies becomes critical. Consider the following strategies:

1. Stockpiling Essential Medications: If you have any prescribed medications, stockpiling them before a crisis is vital. Understand the shelf life of your medications and seek to have a sufficient supply, considering potential alternatives or natural remedies if medications run out.

2. Foraging and Cultivating Medicinal Plants: Familiarize yourself with local flora that can be used for medicinal purposes. Many plants possess healing properties that can help manage chronic conditions. Create a small garden with essential herbs, such as chamomile for anxiety or peppermint for digestive issues.

3. Nutrition and Diet: Focus on a nutrient-rich diet that supports your condition. For example, those with hypertension should prioritize potassium-rich foods like leafy greens and bananas, whereas individuals with arthritis may benefit from omega-3 fatty acids found in fish and walnuts. Learn how to preserve food safely to maintain a balanced diet.

Community Support
In a post-nuclear environment, fostering community ties becomes invaluable. Engage with neighbors and local groups to share resources, knowledge, and support. Consider forming a network of individuals with similar health concerns who can collectively share information, remedies, and emotional support.

Mental and Emotional Resilience
Managing a chronic condition without modern medical support can lead to increased stress and anxiety. Focus on mental resilience by:

1. Practicing Mindfulness: Techniques like meditation and deep-breathing exercises can help lower stress levels and improve emotional well-being.

2. Staying Informed: Knowledge reduces fear. Keep up with reliable information regarding your condition and any available resources in your community.

3. Building a Support Network: Establish connections with others facing similar challenges. Sharing experiences and coping strategies can enhance emotional resilience and provide practical support.

Conclusion
Dealing with chronic conditions in a resource-scarce environment requires adaptability, creativity, and community cooperation. By understanding your illness, creating a personalized management plan, utilizing available resources, and fostering mental resilience, you can navigate the challenges of surviving without modern medicine. With preparation and determination, it is possible to maintain your health and well-being in the face of adversity.

Mental Health Care Post-Attack
In the aftermath of a nuclear attack, the psychological impact can be profound and lasting. Survivors may experience a range of emotional responses, including shock, anxiety, depression, and post-traumatic stress disorder (PTSD). Addressing mental health care in this context is crucial for both individual recovery and community resilience. Here are some strategies to support mental well-being in yourself and others post-attack.

Acknowledge the Impact of Trauma
Recognizing that trauma is a natural response to an extraordinary event is the first step in promoting mental health. Survivors may experience feelings of disbelief, fear, and confusion. Validate these emotions by acknowledging them openly, either through conversation or personal reflection. Encouraging open dialogue about feelings can help alleviate feelings of isolation and stigma.

Create a Supportive Environment
Establishing a supportive environment is essential for mental health recovery. This includes fostering open communication among family members and community members. Share experiences and feelings without judgment. Create safe spaces where individuals feel comfortable expressing their emotions. Encourage group discussions about coping mechanisms and emotional responses, which can help normalize the experience of trauma.

Establish Routines
In chaotic situations, establishing routines can provide a sense of normalcy and stability. Routines can help structure daily life, reducing feelings of uncertainty and anxiety. Simple activities, such as regular meal times, set sleeping hours, and scheduled group discussions, can help individuals regain control over their lives. Encourage participation in these routines, as they can foster a sense of community and belonging.

Implement Coping Strategies
Teaching and encouraging effective coping strategies is vital for emotional resilience. Techniques such as deep breathing exercises, mindfulness, and grounding techniques can help individuals manage anxiety and stress. Practicing these methods can also foster a sense of agency over one's mental state. Encourage journaling as a means of self-reflection, allowing individuals to process their emotions and experiences.

Promote Physical Health
Physical health and mental well-being are interlinked. Encourage survivors to engage in physical activities, which can alleviate stress and improve mood. Simple exercises, such as walking or stretching, can have significant benefits. Additionally, maintaining a balanced diet and ensuring adequate hydration are essential for physical recovery, which in turn supports mental health.

Facilitate Access to Resources
In a post-attack environment, access to professional mental health resources may be limited or nonexistent. Therefore, it is crucial to identify and utilize available resources, such as community leaders, trusted friends, or local support groups. Sharing information about mental health

resources, including potential online support networks, can help survivors find the assistance they need.

Encourage Professional Help When Possible

If circumstances allow, seeking professional help should be encouraged. Mental health professionals can provide specialized support and interventions that aid in recovery. This could include therapy, counseling, or medication management. For those unable to access traditional mental health services, peer support groups can serve as valuable resources for sharing experiences and coping strategies.

Foster a Sense of Purpose

Helping individuals find a sense of purpose in the aftermath of trauma can significantly improve mental health outcomes. Encourage survivors to engage in community rebuilding efforts, volunteer opportunities, or support groups. Focusing on collective recovery can provide hope and a renewed sense of belonging.

Conclusion

The psychological aftermath of a nuclear attack presents unique challenges, but with proactive mental health care and communal support, individuals can navigate their emotional landscapes. By fostering open communication, establishing routines, and promoting coping strategies, communities can facilitate healing and resilience. Ultimately, the journey toward mental well-being is a shared one, and collective efforts can pave the way for recovery and a hopeful future.

The Role of Traditional and Alternative Medicine in a Post-Nuclear World

In the aftermath of a nuclear event, conventional medical infrastructure may be severely compromised or entirely unavailable. Hospitals could be overwhelmed with casualties, while medical supplies may become scarce due to contamination, disruption of supply chains, or an influx of patients suffering from radiation exposure. In such dire circumstances, traditional and alternative medicine can play a vital role in providing care, alleviating suffering, and promoting healing when conventional methods are inaccessible.

Understanding Traditional and Alternative Medicine

Traditional medicine encompasses healing practices that have been passed down through generations, often rooted in the cultural and historical context of a community. This includes herbalism, acupuncture, and various forms of spiritual healing. Alternative medicine refers to practices that are not typically part of conventional medicine and may include homeopathy, naturopathy, and massage therapy. Both approaches can offer valuable insights and remedies, especially in a post-nuclear scenario where immediate medical care may not be available.

Utilizing Herbal Remedies

In the absence of pharmaceutical drugs, herbal remedies can provide effective treatment options for a variety of ailments. Familiarity with local plants and their medicinal properties can be crucial. For instance, herbs such as echinacea and elderberry can boost immune function, while ginger and peppermint can help alleviate digestive issues. Additionally, certain herbs like St. John's Wort may provide relief from symptoms of depression or anxiety, both common in post-disaster scenarios.

When utilizing herbal medicine, it is essential to understand the proper dosages and potential interactions with other remedies. Knowledge of local flora can be enhanced through guides, community knowledge, or even trial and error, but caution should always be exercised to avoid toxic plants.

Acupuncture and Traditional Techniques

Acupuncture, a key component of Traditional Chinese Medicine (TCM), involves inserting fine needles into specific points on the body to promote healing and balance. In a resource-scarce environment, this technique can be beneficial for pain management and stress relief, which are likely to be prevalent in the aftermath of a nuclear event. While practitioners may be hard to find, basic knowledge of acupressure techniques can be applied by individuals to alleviate discomfort without the need for specialized equipment.

Additionally, practices such as yoga and meditation can also help individuals cope with stress and anxiety. These methods promote mental well-being and can be performed with little to no resources, making them accessible to anyone seeking relief in challenging times.

Community-Based Healing Practices

In a post-nuclear society, community-based healing practices can strengthen social ties and foster resilience. Traditional healing rituals, often deeply embedded in cultural identities, can serve as a source of comfort and hope. Community gatherings focused on shared healing practices can help individuals process trauma collectively, reducing feelings of isolation and despair.

Moreover, the exchange of knowledge regarding traditional healing practices can empower communities to be self-reliant. Workshops on foraging for medicinal plants, preparing herbal remedies, or practicing mindfulness can facilitate skill-sharing among community members, enhancing overall resilience.

Ethical Considerations and Limitations

While traditional and alternative medicine offers valuable resources, it is essential to approach these practices with a critical mindset. Not all remedies are effective, and relying solely on unproven methods can lead to adverse outcomes. Combining traditional practices with basic first aid knowledge and, when possible, consulting with trained practitioners remains crucial.

Moreover, understanding the limitations of these practices in the context of severe injuries or acute radiation sickness is vital. In such cases, seeking conventional medical care, if available, should always be prioritized.

Conclusion

In a post-nuclear world, traditional and alternative medicine can provide critical support in maintaining health and well-being when conventional options are limited. By harnessing the knowledge of herbal remedies, community healing practices, and self-care techniques, individuals can cultivate resilience and foster a sense of agency in navigating the challenges of survival.

Chapter 15

Surviving in a New World

Adapting to New Environmental Conditions

In the wake of a nuclear war, the environment will undergo drastic changes. The immediate aftermath may involve widespread devastation, contamination, and a breakdown of societal structures. Adapting to new environmental conditions becomes essential for survival, requiring a multifaceted approach that encompasses physical, psychological, and community-oriented strategies.

Assessing the New Environment

The first step in adapting to a drastically changed environment is a thorough assessment of the new conditions. Survivors must evaluate the immediate landscape for hazards such as radioactive fallout, contaminated water sources, and structural dangers from buildings and infrastructure that may have been damaged or destroyed. Understanding the geography, including the location of safe zones, potential shelters, and areas of contamination, is crucial. Utilizing tools like radiation detectors can help identify safe areas for habitation and resource gathering.

Resource Management

Resource management will be a critical component of survival. Food, water, and shelter will need to be reassessed in light of the new conditions. Survivors should prioritize finding safe water sources, as clean water is essential for survival. Techniques for purifying water, such as boiling or using filtration systems, become vital skills. Additionally, understanding how to identify edible plants and safe food sources in a contaminated environment is crucial. Foraging and hunting may become necessary, and knowledge of local flora and fauna can facilitate this effort.

Shelter Adaptation

Existing shelters may need to be adapted to enhance protection from the elements and potential threats. Survivors should fortify their living spaces against environmental elements, including harsh weather conditions and the risk of radiation exposure. This may involve sealing windows and doors, creating barriers against wind and precipitation, and using available materials to enhance insulation. If possible, constructing a more secure underground shelter or relocating to a less contaminated area can improve safety.

Skills Development

Long-term survival will depend on acquiring new skills that are relevant to the changed environment. This may include learning to cultivate crops in challenging conditions, practicing hunting and trapping techniques, and mastering foraging skills. Knowledge of traditional methods of food preservation, such as drying, fermenting, or canning, can also help extend food supplies. Additionally, skills in first aid and basic medical care will be invaluable, as access to modern medical facilities may be limited or nonexistent.

Mental and Emotional Resilience

Adapting to new environmental conditions also involves addressing the psychological impacts of a drastically changed world. The stress of survival, loss of loved ones, and the uncertainty of the future can lead to anxiety, depression, and other mental health issues. Survivors should develop coping strategies, such as establishing daily routines, engaging in physical activity, and maintaining social connections, even in a challenging environment. Building a sense of community can provide emotional support and foster collaboration in resource sharing and mutual aid.

Building Community and Collaboration

In a post-nuclear world, community becomes a cornerstone of survival. Building networks with other survivors can facilitate resource pooling, skill-sharing, and emotional support. Collaborative efforts, such as forming groups for food production, defense, and education, can significantly enhance the chances of long-term survival. Establishing trust and clear communication within these communities is essential for effective collaboration.

Conclusion

Adapting to new environmental conditions in a post-nuclear world requires resilience, resourcefulness, and a willingness to learn. By assessing the environment, managing resources wisely, developing new skills, maintaining mental health, and building supportive communities, survivors can navigate the challenges they face. The ability to adapt will not only enhance individual survival but also foster the rebuilding of a cohesive, functioning society in the aftermath of catastrophe.

Sustainable Living: Off-Grid Solutions

In a post-nuclear world, where access to modern conveniences may be severely limited or non-existent, learning to live sustainably and off-grid becomes essential for survival. The concept of off-grid living encompasses self-sufficiency in energy, water, food, and waste management, enabling individuals and communities to thrive in a resource-scarce environment.

This section explores practical strategies to achieve sustainable living without relying on traditional infrastructures.

Energy Independence

The first step towards off-grid living is establishing a reliable energy source. Solar power is one of the most viable options for generating electricity in a sustainable manner. Photovoltaic (PV) panels can be installed to harness sunlight, converting it into usable energy. Batteries can be added to store excess energy for use during cloudy days or at night. Additionally, small-scale wind turbines can complement solar energy, particularly in areas with consistent wind patterns. For those living in wooded regions, wood stoves provide heat and can be used for cooking, utilizing sustainably harvested timber.

Water Collection and Purification

Access to clean water is critical for survival. Off-grid living necessitates the collection and purification of water from natural sources. Rainwater harvesting systems can be installed to collect precipitation from roofs, directing it into storage tanks. This water must be filtered and purified before consumption. Techniques such as boiling, UV purification, and charcoal filtration can effectively eliminate contaminants. In regions with rivers or lakes, water can be sourced directly, but it is crucial to use purification methods to ensure safety.

Food Production

Growing food is a cornerstone of sustainable living. Establishing a garden using permaculture principles can maximize yield while minimizing resource input. Raised beds, companion planting, and crop rotation can enhance soil fertility and pest resistance. Additionally, integrating fruit trees, berry bushes, and perennial plants into the landscape creates a diverse food ecosystem. For those with limited space or resources, container gardening is an effective alternative, allowing for food production in small areas.

Foraging is another essential skill in off-grid living. Understanding local flora and fauna can provide access to wild edible plants, nuts, and berries, contributing to a varied diet. It is vital to become educated about which plants are safe to consume and the best times to harvest them.

Waste Management

In an off-grid situation, managing waste becomes critical to maintaining a clean and healthy living environment. Composting organic waste not only reduces waste but also creates nutrient-rich soil for gardens. Compost systems can be as simple as a designated pile or as structured as a bin system. Moreover, implementing a greywater system allows for the reuse of water from sinks and showers for irrigation purposes.

Community Collaboration

While off-grid living emphasizes self-sufficiency, community collaboration plays a crucial role in sustainable living. Forming networks with neighbors can enhance resource sharing, knowledge exchange, and support systems. Bartering goods and services can create a robust local economy that thrives on cooperation rather than reliance on modern conveniences.

Learning and Adaptation

Lastly, embracing a mindset of learning and adaptation is essential for successful off-grid living. Skills such as gardening, animal husbandry, woodworking, and natural building techniques can be invaluable. Workshops, books, and community classes offer opportunities to acquire these skills. Moreover, documenting experiences and sharing knowledge with others fosters resilience and continuity in sustainable living practices.

Living sustainably off-grid not only prepares one for the challenges of a post-nuclear world but also encourages a deeper connection with nature and a more profound respect for resources. By embracing self-sufficiency and community collaboration, individuals can create a thriving ecosystem that supports survival and fosters hope in the face of adversity.

Learning New Skills for Survival

In the wake of a nuclear catastrophe, the ability to adapt becomes paramount for survival. As society breaks down and resources dwindle, acquiring a set of essential skills will not only enhance your chances of survival but also empower you to contribute positively to your community. Here are key skills that will prove invaluable in a post-nuclear environment.

1. Foraging and Wild Food Identification

Understanding how to forage for edible plants, fruits, and nuts is crucial when traditional food sources are unavailable. Familiarize yourself with local flora, focusing on identifying both edible and toxic species. Resources like field guides or apps can help, but practical experience is irreplaceable. Engage with local experts or take classes on wild foraging before a crisis occurs. Remember, the ability to recognize wild food can significantly supplement dwindling food supplies.

2. Basic Agriculture and Gardening

If conditions allow, growing your own food will be vital for long-term survival. Learning the fundamentals of gardening—such as soil preparation, planting techniques, and pest control—will enable you to cultivate crops that can sustain you and your community. Start with fast-growing, resilient plants like radishes, beans, and leafy greens. Understanding crop rotation and companion planting will enhance soil health and yield, ensuring sustainability in your food production.

3. Water Purification Techniques

Access to clean water is essential for survival, particularly in an environment potentially contaminated by radiation or other pollutants. Learn various methods of water purification, such as boiling, filtration, and solar disinfection. Familiarize yourself with natural sources of water, including streams and rainwater collection systems, and understand how to test water for contaminants. Mastering these techniques will ensure you can provide safe drinking water for yourself and others.

4. Basic First Aid and Medical Skills

In a post-nuclear world, access to medical facilities may be limited or nonexistent. Acquiring basic first aid skills, such as wound care, CPR, and the treatment of common injuries and illnesses, will be vital. Consider obtaining certification through a recognized first aid course. Familiarize yourself with the use of herbal remedies and alternative medicine practices, as these may become invaluable when pharmaceutical options are scarce.

5. Self-Defense and Personal Safety

The breakdown of societal norms can lead to increased threats from others. Developing self-defense techniques and situational awareness will enhance your personal safety. Training in martial arts or self-defense classes can provide you with the skills necessary to protect yourself and your loved ones. Additionally, understanding conflict de-escalation strategies can help in navigating potentially hostile encounters, fostering community safety.

6. Fire Creation and Management

Fire is a critical resource for warmth, cooking, and protection. Learn various methods of starting a fire, including using friction, flint and steel, or modern fire starters. Understanding how to build and maintain a fire safely, as well as the importance of firewood preparation, will ensure you can provide warmth and cooked meals. Moreover, fire can serve as a signal for help in emergencies.

7. Crafting and Repairing Skills

In a resource-scarce environment, the ability to repair and craft essential items will be invaluable. Basic skills in sewing, woodworking, and metalworking can allow you to create tools, clothing, and shelter. Learning to repurpose materials can also greatly reduce dependency on external resources, fostering a self-sufficient lifestyle.

Conclusion

The journey toward long-term survival in a post-nuclear world necessitates a proactive approach to learning and skill development. The skills outlined above will not only enhance your chances of survival but also create opportunities for collaboration within your community. By investing time in education and practice, you can build a resilient foundation that promotes sustainability, safety, and community well-being in a drastically changed world.

Reconnecting with Nature: Hunting, Foraging, and Farming

In the aftermath of a nuclear war, the ability to reconnect with nature becomes a vital component of survival. As societal structures crumble and modern conveniences disappear, individuals and communities must learn to depend on natural resources for sustenance. This section explores the essential skills of hunting, foraging, and farming, highlighting how these practices can provide nourishment and foster a deeper connection to the environment.

Hunting: A Timeless Skill for Survival

Hunting is one of the oldest methods of food procurement, and it remains relevant in post-apocalyptic scenarios. To effectively hunt, individuals must develop essential skills, including tracking, understanding animal behavior, and using appropriate tools. Knowledge of local wildlife is crucial; understanding which animals are safe to eat and their seasonal habits can make hunting more successful.

Basic hunting techniques include setting traps, using bows, or firearms where available. Trapping can be advantageous since it allows for passive hunting, freeing individuals to gather other resources while waiting for catches. Additionally, respecting local wildlife laws and ethical hunting practices is vital for maintaining ecological balance. Overhunting can lead to depletion of resources, which can have long-term consequences on local ecosystems.

Foraging: Nature's Bounty

Foraging offers a diverse array of edible plants, fungi, and other natural resources that can supplement or replace traditional food sources. This practice involves identifying wild foods that are safe to consume, which requires knowledge of local flora and fauna. Foragers must learn to recognize edible plants, seasonal variations, and the potential dangers of toxic species.

Common foraged items include wild greens, berries, nuts, and mushrooms. While mushrooms can be nutritious, they also require careful identification, as many varieties are toxic. Field guides and local experts can provide invaluable information for safe foraging practices. Additionally, foraging promotes sustainability by allowing individuals to harvest food without the need for cultivation, thus preserving natural habitats.

Farming: Rebuilding Food Systems

Once immediate survival is secured, cultivating food through farming becomes increasingly essential. In a post-nuclear world, traditional farming practices may need to be adapted to suit the environmental changes resulting from nuclear fallout. Soil contamination and altered ecosystems may pose challenges, but innovative techniques can help overcome these obstacles.

Starting a garden is a practical way to produce food. Growing crops such as potatoes, carrots, and leafy greens can provide essential nutrients. Utilizing raised beds can improve drainage and reduce soil contamination risks. Companion planting—growing different crops together to enhance growth and deter pests—can also be beneficial. Additionally, permaculture principles promote sustainable farming practices that work in harmony with nature, enhancing soil fertility and biodiversity.

In situations where conventional farming is not possible, hydroponics and aquaponics offer alternative methods of food production. These soil-less systems can be set up indoors or in controlled environments, providing fresh produce while minimizing the risk of soil contamination.

Building a Connection with Nature

Reconnecting with nature through hunting, foraging, and farming fosters a deeper appreciation for the environment and its resources. This relationship not only provides sustenance but also promotes mental well-being. Engaging with nature can offer solace and a sense of purpose in the midst of chaos, helping individuals cope with the trauma of a nuclear event.

Moreover, these practices can strengthen community bonds. Collaborating with neighbors in hunting parties, foraging expeditions, or community gardens can enhance social cohesion and resilience. Sharing knowledge and resources fosters a sense of collective responsibility and support, which is essential for long-term survival in a post-nuclear world.

In conclusion, as individuals navigate the challenges of a nuclear aftermath, the skills of hunting, foraging, and farming become indispensable. By relying on nature for food and resources, survivors can not only meet their immediate needs but also lay the foundation for a sustainable future, fostering a renewed relationship with the environment and one another.

The Importance of Community and Collaboration

In the face of cataclysmic events such as a nuclear war, the instinct for self-preservation can often lead individuals to prioritize their own survival over that of others. However, history teaches us that survival in the aftermath of such disasters is not solely an individual endeavor.

The strength of community ties and collaborative efforts can significantly enhance resilience, resourcefulness, and recovery in a post-nuclear world.

The Foundation of Community Resilience

Communities that foster strong relationships are better equipped to navigate crises. When individuals know their neighbors and share mutual trust, they can coordinate efforts to ensure everyone's basic needs are met. This cooperation becomes crucial in the aftermath of a nuclear event, where resources may be scarce, and the threat of radiation and societal breakdown looms. Engaging with one's community before a disaster strikes can help establish a network of support, facilitating resource sharing, communication, and emotional resilience.

Building Trust and Relationships

Trust is the bedrock of any resilient community. Building trust requires consistent interaction, transparency, and the establishment of shared goals. Participating in community activities, such as neighborhood watch programs, local food co-ops, and volunteer initiatives, can foster relationships that will endure during crises. Moreover, organizing preparedness workshops or training sessions can provide community members with the skills they need, while simultaneously strengthening interpersonal bonds.

Collaborative Problem-Solving

In a post-nuclear context, challenges such as food scarcity, water contamination, and health risks will require collective problem-solving. Communities that have practiced collaboration prior to an event will be better suited to tackle these issues. For instance, pooling resources to create a community garden can provide nutritional food, while shared knowledge about water purification methods can ensure safe drinking water. By working together, community members can devise innovative solutions that would be difficult to achieve alone.

Establishing Communication Networks

In the chaos that follows a nuclear event, reliable communication is vital. Establishing a community communication plan can help maintain contact among members and disseminate critical information regarding safety measures, available resources, and recovery efforts. Utilizing radios, bulletin boards, or even designated meeting points can facilitate effective communication, especially when traditional channels are compromised. Communities that prioritize open communication will foster a sense of security and unity, reinforcing their collective strength.

Emotional and Psychological Support

The psychological toll of surviving a nuclear disaster can be immense. Community ties can provide crucial emotional support during these challenging times. Sharing experiences and feelings with others who have faced similar challenges can help mitigate feelings of isolation and despair. Support groups can be established to provide a platform for individuals to express their fears, share coping strategies, and collectively work through trauma. This emotional resilience is as important as physical survival strategies, as mental health plays a significant role in long-term recovery.

Long-Term Sustainability and Adaptation

As communities begin to rebuild, collaboration becomes essential for long-term sustainability. Establishing local governance structures, shared resource management, and community-led initiatives can promote a sense of ownership and responsibility among members. By encouraging local production—whether through community-supported agriculture or cooperative businesses—communities can reduce dependency on external systems that may be unreliable in a post-disaster world.

Conclusion

In conclusion, the importance of community and collaboration in a post-nuclear world cannot be overstated. Strong community ties not only enhance immediate survival prospects but also pave the way for long-term recovery and resilience. By building trust, encouraging collaboration, maintaining communication, and providing emotional support, communities can navigate the complexities of post-disaster life. As individuals come together, they create a collective strength that enables them to face challenges head-on, fostering hope and resilience in the wake of catastrophe. Ultimately, it is this interconnectedness that will help humanity not only survive but thrive in a changed world.

Chapter 16

The Role of Faith and Spirituality

Faith as a Source of Strength and Resilience

In times of catastrophic events, such as a nuclear crisis, the psychological and emotional toll can be overwhelming. Individuals and communities may find themselves grappling with profound loss, fear, and uncertainty about the future. In these tumultuous moments, faith—be it religious or spiritual—can serve as a powerful source of strength and resilience. The role of faith during and after a nuclear crisis encompasses a multitude of aspects that can significantly aid in coping with the aftermath.

Psychological Comfort and Hope

Faith often provides individuals with a fundamental sense of purpose and meaning, which can be crucial during periods of distress. Religious beliefs can offer comforting narratives that help individuals make sense of suffering and loss. For example, many faith traditions include teachings about the value of sacrifice, the promise of renewal, and the hope of life beyond death. These concepts can provide solace, allowing individuals to endure the trauma of a nuclear crisis with a sense of hope for the future. The belief that there is a divine plan, even amid chaos, can help mitigate feelings of despair.

Community Support

Religious communities often act as vital support networks in times of crisis. In the aftermath of a nuclear event, these communities can mobilize quickly to provide emotional, logistical, and spiritual assistance. They may offer food, shelter, and medical aid, creating a safety net for those who are displaced or in need. The communal aspect of faith fosters a sense of belonging, which is essential for psychological well-being. Social connections formed through shared beliefs can also facilitate resilience, as individuals lean on each other for support, encouragement, and practical help.

Rituals and Practices

Faith traditions often include rituals and practices that can play a significant role in coping with trauma. Prayer, meditation, and communal worship can provide individuals with a structured way to process their emotions, seek peace, and find clarity. Engaging in these practices can serve as a form of psychological release, helping individuals to articulate their fears and hopes.

Moreover, rituals can create a sense of normalcy and continuity in the chaotic aftermath of a nuclear crisis, helping individuals re-establish routines that reinforce stability.

Moral Framework
Faith can also provide a moral framework that guides individuals in navigating the ethical dilemmas that may arise in a post-nuclear world. Principles rooted in compassion, empathy, and altruism can help individuals prioritize community needs over individual survival. This moral compass can lead to acts of kindness and cooperation, fostering a spirit of solidarity that is essential for rebuilding society. In a world where resources may be scarce and conflicts may arise, the ethical teachings of faith can encourage collaboration and understanding among survivors.

Coping with Grief and Loss
In the face of loss, faith can be an indispensable tool for coping with grief. Many religious traditions offer specific rites and rituals for mourning, which can help individuals process their emotions in a constructive manner. These practices can create a communal space for expressing sorrow and celebrating the lives of those who have been lost. Furthermore, the belief in an afterlife or a spiritual continuation can provide comfort, allowing individuals to find peace in the face of profound loss.

Conclusion
In summary, faith can serve as a profound source of strength and resilience in the wake of a nuclear crisis. By providing psychological comfort, fostering community support, facilitating coping mechanisms, and offering a moral framework, religious beliefs can help individuals navigate the challenges of survival and recovery. In a post-nuclear world, the power of faith may not only aid individual healing but also play a vital role in rebuilding societies and nurturing hope for future generations. Embracing the strength that faith offers can empower individuals to thrive even amidst the most daunting circumstances.

Spiritual Practices for Coping with Trauma
In the wake of a nuclear war, individuals and communities are likely to face profound psychological trauma, stemming not only from the immediate horrors of destruction and loss but also from the long-term impacts of radiation exposure, societal upheaval, and the uncertainty of rebuilding lives. Spirituality can play a vital role in healing, offering individuals a framework for understanding their experiences, finding meaning amid suffering, and fostering resilience. Here, we explore various spiritual practices that can aid in coping with trauma in the aftermath of a nuclear conflict.

1. Meditation and Mindfulness

Meditation and mindfulness practices can help individuals manage anxiety and stress, which often accompany trauma. These techniques encourage individuals to focus on the present moment, allowing them to observe their thoughts and feelings without judgment. By cultivating a sense of awareness and acceptance, survivors can better navigate the emotional turmoil that follows a nuclear event. Simple mindfulness exercises, such as deep breathing or guided imagery, can be integrated into daily routines, providing moments of peace and clarity amid chaos.

2. Prayer and Reflection

For many, prayer serves as a powerful tool for coping with trauma. Whether through personal reflection or communal prayer, individuals can find solace in expressing their fears, hopes, and desires for healing. This connection to a higher power can foster a sense of support and guidance, alleviating feelings of isolation. Writing in a prayer journal can also facilitate a deeper exploration of one's emotions and thoughts, allowing individuals to process their experiences and articulate their journey toward recovery.

3. Rituals and Ceremonies

Engaging in rituals—whether personal or communal—can provide structure and meaning in the aftermath of chaos. Rituals honoring lost loved ones or marking significant life transitions can help individuals acknowledge their grief and foster a sense of closure. Ceremonies that involve community participation can strengthen social bonds, provide emotional support, and reinforce shared values and beliefs. The act of coming together in a ritualistic manner can combat isolation, creating a collective space for healing.

4. Nature and Spiritual Connection

In the aftermath of a nuclear disaster, reconnecting with nature can be a profound spiritual practice. Nature often symbolizes renewal and resilience, serving as a reminder of life's cyclical nature. Engaging in outdoor activities such as hiking, gardening, or simply spending time in green spaces can promote healing. Many spiritual traditions emphasize the interconnectedness of all life, and spending time in nature can help individuals feel grounded and connected to something larger than themselves.

5. Community and Support Systems

Spirituality is often amplified within a community context. Participating in group activities—be it prayer groups, study circles, or discussion forums—can provide mutual support and shared experiences that foster healing. These gatherings can create a safe space for individuals to express their struggles, fears, and hopes while drawing strength from one another. Community-led initiatives that focus on rebuilding and recovery can instill a sense of purpose and collective resilience.

6. Forgiveness and Letting Go

Healing from trauma often involves the difficult process of forgiveness—whether it be forgiving oneself or others. Spiritual teachings across cultures emphasize the importance of letting go of resentment and anger as a pathway to peace. Engaging in practices that promote forgiveness can free individuals from the burdens of grief and anger, allowing them to move forward with their lives. This can be facilitated through guided meditations focusing on forgiveness or discussions within supportive communities.

Conclusion

In the aftermath of nuclear war, spirituality can serve as a refuge and a source of strength. By incorporating practices such as meditation, prayer, rituals, and community support, individuals can navigate their trauma and cultivate resilience. Spirituality not only offers a means of understanding and processing trauma but also provides hope for rebuilding and restoring a sense of normalcy in an altered world. Through these practices, individuals can forge a path toward healing, fostering both personal and communal recovery.

The Role of Religious Communities in Recovery

In the aftermath of a nuclear catastrophe, the role of religious communities becomes paramount in the recovery and rebuilding process. These groups provide not only spiritual guidance but also practical support, fostering resilience and hope among affected individuals and communities. Their contributions can significantly influence the emotional and physical recovery of survivors, helping to create a cohesive social fabric in the face of unprecedented challenges.

Spiritual Guidance and Emotional Support

Religious communities often serve as primary sources of spiritual solace and emotional support. In times of crisis, faith can be a powerful tool for coping with trauma, grief, and loss. Leaders within these communities, such as clergy and laypersons, can offer counseling and pastoral care, helping individuals process their experiences and emotions. Rituals, prayer services, and memorials can also provide a structured way for community members to grieve collectively, honor lost loved ones, and find solace in their shared beliefs.

Furthermore, religious teachings often emphasize themes of hope, resilience, and community, which can help individuals regain a sense of purpose and direction in their lives. By fostering a sense of belonging and mutual support, faith-based groups can counteract feelings of isolation and despair that may arise in the wake of a nuclear disaster.

Practical Assistance and Resource Distribution

Beyond spiritual support, religious communities are often well-positioned to mobilize resources and provide practical assistance to those in need. Many faith-based organizations have established networks for disaster relief that can be activated quickly in times of crisis. These networks can facilitate the distribution of food, medical supplies, and essential services to affected populations.

For instance, churches, mosques, synagogues, and temples often have established relationships with local and international aid organizations, allowing them to coordinate relief efforts effectively. They can set up shelters, provide meals, and offer psychosocial support to individuals and families struggling to cope with the aftermath of a nuclear event. This ability to mobilize quickly and efficiently can be a lifeline for communities facing the daunting task of recovery.

Building Community Resilience

Religious communities also play a crucial role in building resilience within their neighborhoods. By fostering strong communal ties, these groups can enhance social capital, which is vital during recovery. Faith-based organizations often organize community meetings, workshops, and volunteer initiatives that encourage local engagement and collective problem-solving. By promoting collaboration and solidarity, they help rebuild trust and cooperation among community members, essential for long-term recovery.

Moreover, religious institutions frequently act as advocates for vulnerable populations, ensuring that their voices are heard in the recovery process. They can engage with local governments and aid organizations to address the specific needs of their communities, such as mental health services, housing, and education. This advocacy can be instrumental in shaping recovery policies and ensuring equitable access to resources.

Ethical and Moral Frameworks

In the wake of a nuclear disaster, ethical dilemmas often arise as communities navigate the challenges of survival and recovery. Religious teachings provide moral frameworks that can guide individuals and communities in making difficult decisions. Questions about resource allocation, self-defense, and the treatment of others can be addressed within the context of faith, offering guidance that emphasizes compassion, forgiveness, and community welfare.

Conclusion

In summary, the role of religious communities in recovery after a nuclear event is multifaceted. By providing spiritual guidance, practical assistance, and fostering resilience, these groups can significantly impact the recovery process. Their efforts not only help individuals cope with the immediate aftermath but also lay the groundwork for societal rebuilding, ensuring that hope and solidarity prevail in the face of adversity. As such, acknowledging and supporting the contributions of faith-based groups is essential for fostering recovery and resilience in post-nuclear societies.

Ethical Dilemmas and Moral Decisions

In the aftermath of a nuclear disaster, individuals are likely to confront profound ethical dilemmas that challenge their moral compass and deeply held beliefs. The chaotic environment following such an event—characterized by scarcity of resources, fear, and uncertainty—can lead people to make choices that may conflict with their values. Here, faith and spirituality can play crucial roles in guiding individuals through these tumultuous waters, helping them navigate the complexities of survival while maintaining their humanity.

Navigating Moral Complexities

Survival in a post-nuclear world often involves difficult decisions regarding resource allocation, self-defense, and the treatment of others. For example, one may face the choice of sharing limited food supplies with a neighbor or hoarding them for oneself and one's family. Faith-based teachings emphasizing compassion and altruism can serve as a moral compass, encouraging individuals to prioritize communal well-being over individual gain. In many religious traditions, acts of charity and selflessness are not only encouraged but seen as pathways to spiritual fulfillment and community cohesion.

The Role of Spirituality in Decision-Making

Spiritual beliefs can provide individuals with a framework for understanding the implications of their actions. Spirituality often emphasizes interconnectedness, suggesting that every action has a ripple effect within the community. This understanding can make individuals more aware of the consequences of their choices and promote a sense of responsibility toward others. For instance, someone who believes in a higher moral order may feel compelled to help those who are vulnerable, even at personal risk, because their faith teaches that every life holds inherent value.

Ethical Guidance from Religious Texts

Many religious doctrines contain teachings that can assist in making ethical decisions during crises. For example, the principle of "do no harm" is common across various faiths and can guide individuals in determining how to react when faced with threats, whether from other survivors or from the environment itself. This principle can foster a mindset that seeks non-violent solutions, encouraging negotiation and conflict resolution over aggression.

Compassion as a Survival Strategy

In a post-nuclear world, fostering relationships based on trust and cooperation can be as critical as physical survival strategies. Faith and spirituality often emphasize the importance of community, suggesting that mutual support can enhance resilience. A community that upholds shared values and moral principles may be better equipped to face the challenges of a nuclear aftermath. Those who prioritize compassion may find that building alliances and supporting each other not only aids in survival but also restores a sense of normalcy.

The Challenge of Ethical Decisions under Duress
Despite the guidance offered by faith and spirituality, individuals may still struggle with decisions that pit their survival instincts against their ethical beliefs. For instance, in extreme situations, one might face the temptation to steal or harm others to secure resources. Such actions can lead to guilt and spiritual dissonance, prompting individuals to seek forgiveness or redemption. Faith communities can provide support in these moments, offering counseling, shared experiences, and rituals that help individuals reconcile their actions with their beliefs.

Conclusion: Finding Strength in Faith
Ultimately, faith and spirituality can serve as powerful tools for navigating the ethical dilemmas presented by a post-nuclear world. They help individuals hold onto their humanity, reminding them of the importance of empathy, compassion, and community. While survival may necessitate difficult choices, a strong moral foundation can guide individuals toward actions that honor their values, fostering a sense of hope and purpose in the face of unimaginable challenges. In this way, spirituality not only aids in the navigation of moral complexities but also reinforces the bonds that can lead to collective healing and rebuilding in a fractured world.

Maintaining Hope and Finding Purpose
In the aftermath of a nuclear conflict, individuals face unprecedented challenges that can lead to deep psychological scars, loss of community, and a disconnection from the sense of purpose that once guided their lives. Amidst the chaos and uncertainty, spirituality can serve as a vital anchor, providing a framework for understanding suffering, fostering resilience, and nurturing hope. This section explores how spirituality can assist individuals in maintaining hope and finding purpose in a post-nuclear world.

The Healing Power of Faith
Spiritual beliefs often provide individuals with a sense of meaning that transcends the immediate circumstances of their lives. In times of crisis, many people turn to their faith as a source of comfort and strength. Beliefs about a higher power or the interconnectedness of all life can help individuals reframe their experiences, offering a narrative that instills hope even in the bleakest of situations. This faith can transform despair into a sense of belonging to a larger story, one that encompasses suffering but ultimately leads towards healing and redemption.

Community Support and Shared Beliefs
Spirituality often flourishes in community settings, where shared beliefs and collective practices can foster a sense of solidarity among survivors. In the aftermath of a nuclear event, community support becomes essential. Religious gatherings, whether formal or informal, can serve as safe spaces for individuals to express their fears, share their grief, and find solace in the company of others. This communal aspect of spirituality can reinforce a sense of belonging, reminding

individuals that they are not alone in their struggles. Together, they can engage in rituals, prayers, or meditative practices that promote healing and restoration.

Rituals and Routines: Creating Structure and Meaning
Engaging in spiritual rituals can provide structure and predictability in a chaotic environment. These practices—whether they involve prayer, meditation, or other forms of reflection—can help individuals ground themselves in the present moment. Rituals can act as a reminder of life's continuity and the resilience of the human spirit. They can mark important moments of transition, helping individuals navigate the complexities of their new reality while fostering a sense of purpose.

Finding Meaning in Suffering
Spirituality often encourages individuals to seek meaning in their suffering. Philosophical and theological frameworks, such as those found in many religious traditions, can provide insights into the nature of suffering and the possibility of transformation. This perspective can help survivors see their struggles not as mere tragedies but as opportunities for growth, learning, and deepening their understanding of life. By reframing their experiences, individuals can cultivate a sense of purpose derived from their resilience and capacity to adapt.

Acts of Service and Compassion
In times of crisis, acts of service can become a powerful expression of spirituality. Helping others, whether through community initiatives, sharing resources, or providing emotional support, can foster a sense of purpose and connection. This altruistic behavior reinforces the idea that even in dire circumstances, individuals can contribute positively to the lives of others, creating a ripple effect of hope and resilience. Engaging in service can also provide a sense of agency, allowing survivors to reclaim control over their lives in a world fraught with uncertainty.

Conclusion: Hope as a Collective Endeavor
Ultimately, maintaining hope and finding purpose in a post-nuclear world requires a collective effort. Spirituality can play a crucial role in this process, offering individuals the tools to navigate their experiences while nurturing connections with others. By fostering faith, community bonds, rituals, and acts of compassion, spirituality can transform despair into hope, guiding individuals toward a renewed sense of purpose in the aftermath of tragedy. In this way, the human spirit can rise from the ashes, resilient and determined to rebuild a meaningful existence amidst the ruins.

Chapter 17

Government and Authority in Post-Nuclear Society

The Role of Government in Crisis Management

In the context of nuclear threats, the role of government in crisis management is multifaceted and critical to ensuring national safety and public resilience. Governments bear the responsibility of preparing for potential nuclear incidents through comprehensive planning, coordination, and communication strategies. This preparation encompasses a wide range of activities, from policy formulation and military readiness to public education and emergency response mechanisms.

Policy Formulation and Legal Framework

Governments must establish a robust legal and policy framework to address nuclear threats effectively. This includes international treaties aimed at non-proliferation, disarmament, and the peaceful use of nuclear energy, such as the Treaty on the Non-Proliferation of Nuclear Weapons (NPT). Domestically, governments often enact legislation that outlines the powers and responsibilities of various agencies in the event of a nuclear crisis. These laws typically empower emergency management authorities, health departments, and public safety agencies to coordinate their responses effectively.

Intelligence and Threat Assessment

An essential aspect of government preparedness involves the continuous monitoring of global nuclear activities. Intelligence agencies play a pivotal role in assessing threats from nuclear-armed states or non-state actors. By analyzing satellite imagery, intercepting communications, and engaging in diplomatic channels, governments can gauge the intentions and capabilities of potential adversaries. This intelligence informs policymakers, allowing them to take preemptive actions, engage in diplomatic negotiations, or prepare for possible military responses.

Emergency Preparedness and Response Planning

Governments invest heavily in emergency preparedness and response planning to mitigate the impact of a nuclear incident. This includes the development of comprehensive emergency response plans that detail the roles of various agencies in the event of a nuclear attack. Such plans typically encompass evacuation protocols, sheltering strategies, and medical response frameworks. Regular drills and simulations are conducted to test these plans and ensure that first responders and emergency personnel are equipped to handle the complexities of a nuclear crisis.

Public Education and Awareness Campaigns
An informed public is a crucial component of effective crisis management. Governments are responsible for educating citizens about nuclear threats and the appropriate actions to take during an incident. Public awareness campaigns often include information on recognizing warning signs, understanding the importance of sheltering, and knowing how to access emergency services. These campaigns aim to empower individuals and communities, enhancing their resilience in the face of potential nuclear threats.

Coordination with Local and International Partners
Crisis management in the context of a nuclear threat requires seamless coordination among various government levels and agencies. Federal, state, and local governments must work together to ensure that resources are allocated efficiently and that communication remains open during a crisis. Additionally, international cooperation is vital. Governments often collaborate with global organizations, such as the United Nations and the International Atomic Energy Agency (IAEA), to share intelligence, resources, and best practices for nuclear threat mitigation.

Resource Allocation and Infrastructure
Effective crisis management necessitates the allocation of resources for infrastructure that can withstand nuclear incidents. This includes building and maintaining fallout shelters, ensuring that critical facilities (such as hospitals and emergency operation centers) are equipped to handle radiation exposure, and investing in technologies for radiation detection and decontamination. Governments must also prioritize the training of personnel who will be tasked with managing nuclear emergencies.

Conclusion
In summary, the role of government in crisis management regarding nuclear threats is comprehensive and involves proactive preparedness, effective response planning, public education, and international cooperation. By establishing a well-coordinated framework, governments can enhance national security and safeguard public health during times of crisis, ultimately fostering resilience in the face of potentially catastrophic nuclear events.

Martial Law and Civil Liberties: What to Expect
In the aftermath of a nuclear attack, the imposition of martial law may become a crucial and immediate necessity for governments attempting to manage chaos and restore order. Martial

law involves the temporary suspension of normal civil rights and the application of military authority to enforce laws. This drastic measure can arise from the need to protect public safety, maintain order, and provide essential services during a crisis. Understanding its implications is vital for individuals and communities preparing for such scenarios.

The Nature of Martial Law

Martial law typically entails the military taking over the functions of civilian government. This can include the enforcement of curfews, restrictions on movement, and the prohibition of gatherings. Law enforcement agencies may be augmented by military personnel, and the usual judicial processes may be suspended. In extreme cases, the legal system can operate under military tribunals instead of civilian courts, leading to expedited justice that may bypass traditional legal protections.

The rationale behind martial law is the belief that in times of extreme threat—such as the aftermath of a nuclear explosion—swift, decisive actions are necessary to prevent anarchy and ensure public safety. The government might argue that the extraordinary circumstances justify the suspension of certain civil liberties, aiming to restore a semblance of normalcy as quickly as possible.

Implications for Civil Liberties

The imposition of martial law can significantly impact civil liberties, including:

1. Freedom of Movement: Citizens may experience restrictions on their ability to travel within and outside designated areas. Checkpoints may be established, and individuals could be required to present identification or permits to move freely.

2. Right to Assemble: Public gatherings may be banned to prevent riots or civil disturbances. This restriction can hinder the ability of communities to organize, protest, or share information.

3. Freedom of Speech: Censorship may occur as the government seeks to control the narrative and prevent panic. Media outlets might face restrictions on reporting certain information, particularly details about the government's response or military operations.

4. Due Process: The right to a fair trial could be compromised under martial law. Arrests may occur without warrants, and legal representation might not be guaranteed, leading to potential abuses of power.

5. Privacy Rights: Surveillance measures might increase significantly as the military and law enforcement agencies monitor communications and movements to preempt potential threats. This can lead to a loss of personal privacy.

The Psychological Impact
The psychological ramifications of martial law can be profound. Citizens may experience heightened anxiety and fear due to the uncertainty surrounding their rights and the actions of those in power. The loss of civil liberties can lead to feelings of helplessness and distrust in authorities. Communities may fracture as individuals grapple with conflicting loyalties between following directives and preserving personal freedoms.

Preparing for Martial Law
For individuals and communities, understanding the potential for martial law necessitates preparedness. It is essential to stay informed about government protocols and develop communication networks to share information. Establishing a clear understanding of rights—even under martial law—can empower individuals to advocate for themselves and their communities.

Moreover, fostering community solidarity can provide a support system during times of uncertainty. Engaging in discussions about ethical considerations and the balance between security and liberty can also help communities navigate the complexities of martial law, ensuring that voices are heard even in the face of potential oppression.

Conclusion
Martial law represents a challenging intersection of security and liberty that must be navigated carefully in the wake of a nuclear event. While the intent may be to maintain order and protect citizens, the implications for civil liberties can be profound and lasting. Awareness, preparedness, and community resilience will be crucial in facing these challenges head-on, ensuring that the values of democracy and human rights are upheld even in the most trying circumstances.

The Importance of Law and Order in Survival
In the aftermath of a nuclear war, the immediate focus for survivors shifts from the chaos of destruction to the establishment of a functional society capable of supporting its members. Maintaining law and order is not merely a matter of governance; it is a cornerstone of survival that influences every aspect of life in a post-nuclear environment. The breakdown of societal structures following a catastrophic event can lead to chaos, violence, and a struggle for

resources, which can further jeopardize the chances of survival for individuals and communities alike.

Restoration of Social Cohesion
Law and order serve as the framework for social cohesion, which is crucial in the wake of a nuclear disaster. In times of crisis, people often look for leadership and structure. A functional legal system can provide a sense of normalcy and predictability, essential for reducing anxiety and fostering cooperation among survivors. When the rule of law is upheld, individuals are more likely to engage in collective efforts to rebuild society, share resources, and support one another. In this context, law enforcement and community leaders play a vital role in mediating conflicts, ensuring equitable resource distribution, and maintaining peace.

Protection of Vulnerable Populations
A breakdown of law and order can lead to the victimization of vulnerable populations, including women, children, and the elderly. In the absence of legal protections, these groups are at a heightened risk of exploitation and violence. Establishing a legal framework and community support systems is essential to safeguard the rights and well-being of all individuals. This entails not only the enforcement of laws but also the creation of community watch groups and support networks that can offer protection and assistance to those most at risk.

Resource Management and Conflict Prevention
Scarcity of resources—such as food, water, and medical supplies—inevitably arises in the aftermath of a nuclear event. This scarcity can lead to desperation and conflict among survivors. A well-established law and order system can help manage these resources effectively, preventing hoarding, theft, and violence. Clear guidelines and rules regarding resource allocation and usage can mitigate potential conflicts. Furthermore, a functioning legal system can facilitate negotiations and agreements among groups, ensuring that resources are shared equitably and sustainably.

Restoration of Infrastructure and Services
The restoration of essential services—such as healthcare, transportation, and utilities—requires a stable and organized approach. Law and order are fundamental to the coordination of recovery efforts. Government and local authorities must be able to manage restoration projects efficiently, which involves not only rebuilding physical infrastructure but also reinstating public trust in the institutions responsible for governance. Without law and order, these efforts can become disorganized, leading to delays and further frustration within the community.

Psychological Stability and Community Resilience

The psychological impacts of surviving a nuclear event can be profound, leading to trauma, anxiety, and a sense of hopelessness. The presence of law and order can provide psychological stability by establishing a predictable environment in which individuals can begin to heal and rebuild their lives. When communities feel safe and supported by a functioning legal system, they are more likely to foster social bonds and resilience, which are essential for long-term recovery.

Conclusion

In the wake of a nuclear catastrophe, maintaining law and order is crucial not only for immediate survival but also for the long-term recovery and rebuilding of society. The rule of law fosters social cohesion, protects the vulnerable, manages resources, restores infrastructure, and provides psychological stability. It is essential for survivors to understand the importance of governance, collective responsibility, and community support in overcoming the challenges posed by such a devastating event. A well-ordered society can lay the foundation for a hopeful future, fostering resilience and unity in the face of adversity.

The Role of International Organizations in Post-Nuclear Scenarios

In the aftermath of a nuclear event, the role of international organizations becomes critical in managing the multifaceted challenges that arise. These organizations, including the United Nations (UN), the World Health Organization (WHO), and the International Atomic Energy Agency (IAEA), each play unique roles that can facilitate recovery, provide humanitarian aid, and promote global stability. Understanding how these entities can intervene and assist is essential for comprehending the broader implications of nuclear warfare and the pathways to recovery.

Humanitarian Assistance and Disaster Relief

One of the primary roles of international organizations in post-nuclear scenarios is to coordinate humanitarian assistance and disaster relief. The UN, through its various agencies, can mobilize resources quickly to provide food, water, medical supplies, and shelter to affected populations. The UN's Office for the Coordination of Humanitarian Affairs (OCHA) is specifically responsible for coordinating international humanitarian responses, ensuring that aid reaches those in need efficiently and effectively. This includes setting up logistics for transporting supplies, establishing temporary shelters, and deploying medical teams to address immediate health concerns resulting from the nuclear event.

Health Response and Radiation Management

The WHO plays a pivotal role in addressing health crises following a nuclear explosion. The organization can provide essential guidance on managing radiation exposure and treating radiation sickness. It can also help in setting up health infrastructure to deal with acute medical emergencies and long-term health monitoring. The WHO can deploy experts to assess health needs, manage disease outbreaks, and develop public health strategies tailored to the unique challenges of a nuclear-impacted environment. Furthermore, they can assist in training local healthcare providers to handle the specific needs of radiation-related health issues.

Nuclear Safety and Security Oversight

The IAEA's involvement is crucial in the context of nuclear safety and security. Following a nuclear attack, the agency can assess the status of nuclear facilities, provide expert advice on decontamination processes, and help prevent further nuclear incidents. The IAEA is also responsible for ensuring that any nuclear materials are secured to prevent illicit trafficking or further proliferation. Their role extends to facilitating the safe disposal of radioactive waste and advising on long-term environmental recovery strategies.

Political Mediation and Conflict Resolution

International organizations also serve as mediators in the geopolitical tensions that may arise post-nuclear conflict. The UN can facilitate dialogue among nations to prevent escalation into further violence. Through diplomatic channels and peacekeeping missions, the UN can help stabilize regions affected by nuclear war, fostering an environment conducive to rebuilding and reconciliation. This is especially important in preventing retaliatory strikes or escalation through misunderstandings that could arise from the chaotic aftermath of a nuclear event.

Building Resilience and Promoting Disarmament

Beyond immediate response efforts, international organizations play a long-term role in promoting resilience and disarmament. The UN, through various treaties and initiatives, works toward nuclear disarmament and non-proliferation. In a post-nuclear context, these efforts become even more vital, as the world grapples with the lessons learned and strives to prevent future conflicts. Organizations can facilitate international cooperation to strengthen treaties and agreements that deter nuclear weapons use, fostering a global security environment that prioritizes peace and stability.

Conclusion

In summary, international organizations are indispensable in the aftermath of a nuclear event. Their multifaceted roles, from humanitarian aid and health management to safety oversight and political mediation, provide a framework for recovery and resilience. By leveraging their resources, expertise, and diplomatic channels, these organizations can help mitigate the immediate impacts of nuclear disasters and pave the way for long-term recovery and global disarmament efforts. As the world navigates the complex landscape of nuclear threats, the importance of these organizations cannot be overstated; they serve as beacons of hope and cooperation in a fractured world.

Preparing for Potential Government Failures

In a post-nuclear world, the failure of government structures and services poses significant risks to survival. The sudden disruption of authority can lead to chaos, lack of essential services, and a breakdown of social order. Therefore, preparedness is essential for individuals and communities to navigate such crises effectively.

Understanding the Risks of Government Failure

Governments may fail or become incapacitated due to a nuclear event for several reasons: physical destruction of infrastructure, communication breakdown, mass panic, and resource scarcity. In such scenarios, individuals must recognize that reliance on government support will be limited, necessitating proactive measures to ensure personal and community survival.

Developing a Self-Sufficient Mindset

To prepare for potential government failures, cultivating a self-sufficient mindset is crucial. This involves understanding that individuals will need to rely on their resources, skills, and community networks. Encourage self-education on survival skills, including basic first aid, food foraging, water purification, and self-defense. Recognizing that you may need to take charge of your own survival will empower you to act decisively in times of crisis.

Building Community Networks

Strong community ties are vital during government failures. Collaborate with neighbors to establish a mutual aid network, where members agree to share resources, skills, and information. Forming alliances can enhance security, facilitate resource sharing, and provide emotional support. Regularly meeting to discuss preparedness plans and conducting drills can foster a sense of unity and readiness within the community.

Stockpiling Essential Supplies

In anticipation of government failure, individuals should stockpile essential supplies. This includes non-perishable food, water, medical supplies, and other necessities. Consider creating a "bug-out bag" containing critical items that can be quickly accessed if you need to evacuate. Supplies should be rotated regularly to ensure freshness, and it's wise to plan for a minimum of several weeks' worth of provisions.

Establishing Communication Channels

With potential disruptions to traditional communication systems, establishing alternative channels is essential. Invest in hand-crank or solar-powered radios to receive updates. Set up a system of signals or meetings with your community to share information. If possible, learn about amateur radio (HAM radio) as a means of communication when other systems fail.

Developing a Security Plan

With government structures in disarray, personal safety becomes paramount. Create a comprehensive security plan that includes home fortification strategies and self-defense training. Assess your immediate environment for vulnerabilities and consider how to secure your shelter against potential threats. Establish protocols for responding to unwanted encounters and ensure that everyone in your household understands these procedures.

Creating a Plan for Resource Management

In the absence of government support, managing resources becomes critical. Develop a strategy for rationing supplies, especially food and water. Engage in discussions with your community about shared resources and how to prioritize their use. This collective approach can help extend the lifespan of supplies and enhance overall resilience.

Mental and Emotional Preparedness

The psychological impact of government failure can be profound. Stress, anxiety, and fear may arise in such uncertain times. Developing mental resilience is just as important as physical preparedness. Techniques such as mindfulness, meditation, and open communication with loved ones can help manage stress. Encourage community discussions about mental health and coping strategies to foster a supportive environment.

Conclusion

Preparing for potential government failures in a post-nuclear world requires foresight, adaptability, and community collaboration. By cultivating a self-sufficient mindset, building strong community networks, stockpiling supplies, and developing comprehensive plans for security and resource management, individuals can enhance their chances of survival. Mental resilience and emotional support will be critical in navigating the challenges ahead. With these preparations in place, individuals can approach the uncertain future with greater confidence and determination.

Chapter 18

Ethics and Morality in Survival Situations

The Ethics of Survival: Difficult Decisions

In the harrowing aftermath of a nuclear catastrophe, individuals are thrust into extreme survival situations that challenge not only their physical endurance but also their moral compass. The ethics of survival in such contexts become profoundly complex, as decisions must be made that can weigh heavily on the conscience and challenge deeply held values. Navigating these moral complexities requires both introspection and an understanding of the broader implications of one's choices.

At the heart of ethical decision-making during a survival scenario is the principle of self-preservation versus the needs of the community. In dire situations, individuals often face choices that pit their survival against the welfare of others. For example, when resources such as food, water, or medical supplies are scarce, the instinct to prioritize one's own survival can conflict with the desire to help others. This dilemma raises critical questions: Is it justifiable to take resources from others for one's survival? Should one share limited supplies, risking their own life for the sake of others?

In addressing these questions, it is vital to consider the concept of reciprocity and community reliance. Human beings are inherently social creatures, and fostering a sense of community can be essential for survival. Collaborative efforts often lead to better outcomes than solitary ones, as pooling resources can enhance the chances of survival for all involved. Therefore, while self-preservation is instinctual, it is equally important to weigh the impact of one's actions on the collective. Compassion and cooperation may not only save lives but can also reinforce moral integrity and community bonds.

Another ethical consideration is the potential for violence and coercion. In desperate situations, the breakdown of societal norms can lead to an environment where individuals may resort to theft, violence, or exploitation. The choice to engage in such behaviors poses serious ethical dilemmas. One must consider the long-term implications of these actions, not just for personal survival but for the moral fabric of any remaining community. Engaging in violence may provide short-term gains but can lead to long-lasting distrust and resentment, ultimately undermining any chance of collective recovery.

Furthermore, the ethics of survival also encompass the treatment of vulnerable populations—children, the elderly, and the sick. Decisions regarding who receives care and support can be particularly challenging. For instance, in a scenario where medical resources are limited, a caregiver may face the heart-wrenching choice of allocating scarce medical supplies to those most likely to survive or to those who are most vulnerable. Ethical frameworks such as utilitarianism, which advocates for the greatest good for the greatest number, can provide guidance, yet they can also lead to difficult moral trade-offs that weigh heavily on decision-makers.

Additionally, individuals may grapple with the ethical implications of their survival strategies. Decisions about how to hunt, gather, or scavenge resources can bring about ethical questions related to environmental stewardship and sustainability. Exploiting resources without consideration can lead to long-term ecological damage, which may hinder future survival prospects for both individuals and communities.

In conclusion, the ethics of survival in extreme conditions demand a nuanced approach to decision-making that balances self-preservation with community welfare. Engaging with moral complexities requires individuals to reflect on their values and the potential consequences of their actions. By fostering compassion, cooperation, and a sense of shared responsibility, survivors can navigate the treacherous waters of ethical dilemmas while preserving both their humanity and the hope for a more sustainable future in a post-catastrophe world.

Balancing Self-Preservation and Community Needs

In the aftermath of a nuclear event, individuals face the profound challenge of balancing their instinct for self-preservation with the needs of the community. This delicate equilibrium is vital for not only survival but also the rebuilding of social structures that may be severely disrupted. Understanding how to navigate this balance requires a nuanced approach that incorporates ethical considerations, practical strategies, and psychological resilience.

Understanding the Instincts

Self-preservation is a fundamental human instinct that drives individuals to seek safety, food, and shelter. In a post-nuclear world, this instinct may manifest as hoarding resources, isolating from others, or prioritizing personal safety over communal well-being. While these behaviors can be seen as natural reactions to extreme stress and uncertainty, they can also lead to social fragmentation and increased tensions within communities.

Conversely, the needs of the community—safety, cooperation, and mutual support—are essential for collective survival. A strong community can provide emotional support, share resources, and enhance security against external threats. This interconnectedness is crucial in overcoming the psychological and physical challenges posed by a nuclear disaster.

Ethical Considerations

Balancing self-preservation with community needs often involves navigating ethical dilemmas. Individuals may be faced with difficult decisions regarding resource allocation, where they must choose between their well-being and that of others. Ethical frameworks, such as utilitarianism (maximizing overall happiness) or deontological ethics (adhering to moral rules), can guide these decisions. For instance, one might prioritize sharing food with a family in need over personal stockpiling, recognizing that a healthy community increases the chances of survival for everyone.

Practical Strategies

1. Resource Sharing: Establishing a system for sharing resources can prevent hoarding and promote trust. Community members can organize food banks or communal shelters, where individuals contribute what they can and receive help in return. This fosters a sense of belonging and mutual reliance.

2. Collaborative Decision-Making: In a post-nuclear environment, collective decision-making can help balance individual and community needs. Creating councils or committees can ensure that everyone's voice is heard, allowing for more equitable resource distribution and conflict resolution.

3. Education and Training: Providing community members with training in survival skills—such as first aid, foraging, and self-defense—empowers individuals while enhancing community resilience. When people feel capable and knowledgeable, they are more likely to contribute positively to group efforts.

4. Open Communication: Establishing clear communication channels fosters transparency and trust. Regular meetings or check-ins can help address concerns, share knowledge, and plan for collective strategies, ensuring that everyone is invested in the community's success.

5. Emotional Support Systems: In the wake of trauma, people will experience a range of emotions, from fear to grief. Building support networks where individuals can share their feelings and experiences is crucial for mental health. This communal healing can reinforce bonds and encourage cooperative behavior.

Psychological Resilience

The psychological impact of a nuclear disaster can lead to feelings of isolation and despair. Recognizing this, individuals should cultivate resilience not just for themselves but also for their communities. Encouraging acts of kindness, empathy, and collaboration can create a positive feedback loop that benefits both individual and community survival.

Ultimately, the balance between self-preservation and community needs is not a zero-sum game. By fostering an environment where individuals feel safe to contribute and support one another, communities can enhance their collective resilience and increase the chances of long-term survival. In a world where the threat of nuclear conflict looms large, this balance becomes not only a survival strategy but a pathway to rebuilding a more interconnected and compassionate society.

The Role of Compassion and Humanity

In the grim reality of a post-nuclear war world, survival instincts may push individuals towards self-preservation at the expense of community. However, maintaining empathy and compassion is not only a moral imperative but also a practical necessity for the long-term survival of individuals and communities. The capacity for compassion can enhance social cohesion, improve psychological resilience, and ultimately foster environments conducive to recovery and rebuilding.

The Importance of Compassion in Crisis

Compassion serves as a powerful antidote to fear and despair. In the aftermath of a nuclear disaster, people will undoubtedly experience a range of intense emotions, including shock, grief, and anxiety. During these turbulent times, acts of kindness and support can create a sense of hope and connection. Studies have shown that communities that exhibit strong social bonds are better equipped to recover from disasters, as they can pool resources, share knowledge, and provide emotional support to one another.

Moreover, compassion can mitigate the psychological impacts of trauma. In a survival situation, individuals might witness or experience profound suffering. Being able to empathize with others and extend help can foster a sense of purpose and agency, counteracting feelings of helplessness. Compassionate actions—whether it's sharing food, providing medical assistance, or simply offering a listening ear—can enhance mental well-being for both the giver and the receiver.

Practicing Compassion in Survival Situations

1. Cultivating Empathy: Empathy involves understanding and sharing the feelings of others. Practicing active listening and putting oneself in another's shoes can help individuals connect emotionally, even in dire situations. Sharing stories, discussing fears, and expressing feelings can build trust and understanding, reinforcing community bonds.

2. Shared Resources: In a resource-scarce environment, the instinct may be to hoard supplies. However, sharing resources can foster interdependence and mutual support. Establishing communal kitchens, first-aid stations, or shared shelter spaces can facilitate cooperation. Individuals should be encouraged to contribute whatever they can, reinforcing the idea that collective survival benefits everyone.

3. Creating Support Networks: Forming support groups can help individuals process their emotions and experiences. These networks can serve as platforms for sharing information, resources, and emotional support. Regular meetings can provide a sense of normalcy and community, which is essential for mental health in a chaotic environment.

4. Encouraging Altruism: Altruistic behavior often enhances the psychological well-being of the helper. Engaging in acts of kindness, whether big or small, can help individuals feel more connected and less isolated. Encouraging community members to volunteer their time and skills for collective efforts can forge strong ties and enhance the overall resilience of the group.

5. Leading by Example: Those in leadership roles—whether formal or informal—should model compassionate behavior. Demonstrating empathy and prioritizing the well-being of the community can inspire others to act similarly. Leaders should create an environment where compassion is recognized and valued, reinforcing its importance in survival.

The Long-Term Benefits of Compassion
In a post-nuclear world, the challenges of survival will require not just physical resources but also emotional and social resilience. Compassion and humanity can drive collaborative efforts for recovery, help restore a sense of normalcy, and foster environments where healing can take place. By prioritizing empathy, individuals can not only enhance their chances of survival but also contribute to the rebuilding of a more compassionate society.

Ultimately, in the face of catastrophic events, it is humanity's capacity for compassion that can illuminate the darkest paths, guiding communities toward recovery, resilience, and a hopeful future.

Legal and Ethical Challenges in Post-Nuclear Society
In the aftermath of a nuclear event, society will face an unprecedented array of legal and ethical challenges that will shape the fabric of human interaction and governance. The catastrophic consequences of nuclear warfare will necessitate urgent decision-making in contexts where laws may be rendered obsolete, and moral compasses can become disoriented under extreme stress. Understanding these challenges is crucial for individuals and communities preparing for a post-nuclear world.

1. Legal Frameworks and Governance

One of the primary challenges in a post-nuclear society will be the erosion or complete breakdown of existing legal frameworks. With the potential for widespread destruction and loss of life, local, state, and national governments may struggle to maintain order and provide governance. The imposition of martial law may become necessary to restore some semblance of societal structure. However, this can lead to significant ethical dilemmas regarding civil liberties. Individuals may face curfews, restrictions on movement, and even detainment without due process, raising questions about the balance between security and personal freedoms.

Furthermore, the enforcement of laws may become inconsistent or entirely reliant on the authority of military or paramilitary groups, leading to potential abuses of power. The lack of a functioning legal system creates an environment ripe for corruption, exploitation, and violence, complicating the establishment of a just society.

2. Resource Allocation and Scarcity

In a post-nuclear world, resources such as food, water, and medical supplies will be scarce. This scarcity presents ethical dilemmas about how to allocate these critical resources. Questions will arise regarding who gets access to limited supplies: Should it be based on need, contribution to community survival, or first-come, first-served? The decisions made in these moments can lead to significant moral conflicts, as individuals may be forced to prioritize family over community or vice versa.

Additionally, the potential for hoarding or black market activities will challenge existing laws and ethical norms. Communities may need to grapple with whether to enforce communal sharing of resources or allow individuals to operate freely, risking further inequality and conflict.

3. Self-Defense and Security

As societal structures break down, personal security will become a pressing concern. Individuals and communities may feel compelled to take up arms for protection. This raises complex legal questions regarding self-defense and the use of lethal force. What constitutes legitimate self-defense in a lawless environment? How can communities establish rules of engagement to prevent escalating violence? The moral implications of defending oneself or others, especially in situations where innocent lives may be at risk, will require careful consideration and dialogue within communities.

4. Moral Dilemmas and Community Relations

Survivors will face moral dilemmas that can fracture community bonds. Decisions regarding the treatment of outsiders, perceived enemies, or individuals who have violated societal norms will test the limits of compassion and justice. The ethical principle of "survival of the fittest" may tempt some to abandon ethical considerations in favor of self-preservation, leading to potential violence against those deemed 'other.'

Moreover, the question of rehabilitation versus punishment for those who committed crimes during the chaos will challenge communities. Balancing the need for justice against the necessity of rebuilding trust and social cohesion will be a significant ethical hurdle.

5. Reimagining Justice
Ultimately, the legal and ethical challenges in a post-nuclear society will require a reimagining of justice. Traditional legal systems may not suffice, prompting the need for restorative justice practices that emphasize healing and community rebuilding over punitive measures. This approach could foster dialogue and facilitate a path toward reconciliation in a fractured society.

In conclusion, the legal and ethical dilemmas that will emerge in a post-nuclear world are complex and multifaceted. As individuals and communities prepare for the potential realities of nuclear conflict, cultivating a deep understanding of these challenges is vital for fostering resilience, justice, and humanity in the aftermath of catastrophe.

Preparing for Ethical Challenges: Moral Readiness
In the context of a post-nuclear war environment, the moral landscape can become profoundly complex. The decisions individuals make in such dire circumstances often carry significant ethical weight, demanding a preparedness that goes beyond physical survival. Mental and emotional readiness for ethical challenges is crucial for sustaining not only personal integrity but also the fabric of any remaining community. Here, we explore strategies for enhancing moral readiness in the face of extreme adversity.

Understanding the Ethical Landscape
To mentally prepare for the moral challenges of survival, it is essential first to understand the ethical landscape that may arise. This landscape is fraught with dilemmas that pit self-preservation against the needs of others. For instance, when resources become scarce—food, water, or shelter—individuals may be faced with difficult choices about sharing with others or hoarding supplies for their own safety. Recognizing that these dilemmas will likely occur can help individuals brace themselves for the moral weight of such decisions.

Developing a Personal Ethical Framework
One effective way to prepare for potential moral challenges is to develop a personal ethical framework ahead of time. This framework should reflect one's values and principles, providing guidelines for decision-making during crises. Questions to consider include: What are my non-negotiable values? How do I define fairness and justice? What role does compassion play in my survival strategy?

By contemplating these questions beforehand, individuals can create a moral compass that can guide their decisions during stressful situations. This framework can also help to mitigate feelings of guilt or remorse that may arise after making tough choices, as individuals can refer back to their established principles.

Engaging in Ethical Reflection and Dialogue

Engaging in discussions about hypothetical survival scenarios with friends, family, or community members can also enhance moral readiness. These dialogues allow individuals to explore various perspectives and ethical considerations, fostering a deeper understanding of the complexities of survival ethics. Role-playing different scenarios can provide insights into how one might react under pressure, revealing personal biases and encouraging empathy for others' situations.

Practicing Empathy and Compassion

In a survival situation, it can be easy to become self-focused, leading to a breakdown of community ties and social cohesion. Practicing empathy and compassion, even in lesser stressful situations, can prepare individuals for the emotional challenges of a post-nuclear world. This practice involves actively considering the feelings and needs of others. Engaging in volunteer work or community service prior to a crisis can cultivate a sense of social responsibility that may carry over into a survival context.

Maintaining Moral Flexibility

While it is essential to have a personal ethical framework, it is equally important to maintain a degree of moral flexibility. The unpredictability of survival scenarios may require individuals to adapt their ethical considerations to the realities they face. For example, the urgency of saving a life may outweigh the considerations of resource sharing. Embracing the idea that ethics can be context-dependent allows individuals to navigate dilemmas with a nuanced understanding of right and wrong.

Final Thoughts: Building Moral Resilience

Ultimately, moral readiness is about building resilience in the face of ethical challenges. This involves not only preparation but also ongoing self-reflection and a commitment to maintaining one's humanity amidst chaos. By fostering a strong ethical foundation, engaging in thoughtful dialogue, practicing empathy, and embracing moral flexibility, individuals can navigate the treacherous waters of survival with integrity and compassion. In doing so, they can contribute to the rebuilding of a society that values not just survival, but also the humane treatment of all its members.

Chapter 19

Learning from History

Hiroshima and Nagasaki

The atomic bombings of Hiroshima and Nagasaki in August 1945 remain pivotal moments in history, not only due to their immediate catastrophic effects but also because of the profound lessons they impart regarding nuclear warfare and its aftermath. Survivors, known as hibakusha, have shared their experiences, shedding light on the physical, psychological, and societal ramifications of living through such unprecedented devastation.

Understanding the Immediate Impact

The immediate effects of the atomic bombs were catastrophic. In Hiroshima, the bomb, known as "Little Boy," detonated on August 6, 1945, with a force equivalent to approximately 15 kilotons of TNT. The explosion obliterated around 70,000 buildings and killed an estimated 140,000 people by the end of the year, with many more suffering from severe burns and radiation sickness. In Nagasaki, the bomb, "Fat Man," detonated three days later, claiming an estimated 70,000 lives and causing similar destruction. Survivors reported a blinding flash of light followed by an intense heatwave, which incinerated everything within a certain radius, leaving a haunting landscape of desolation.

Psychological and Emotional Resilience

The psychological impact on survivors was profound and long-lasting. Many hibakusha faced not only the trauma of the event itself but also the stigma associated with radiation exposure, which often led to social isolation. Survivors reported feelings of guilt, particularly those who had lost loved ones or who had been unable to help others. The importance of mental health care and community support emerged as critical themes in their narratives. Survivors emphasized the need for emotional resilience, highlighting the significance of sharing their stories and experiences as a means of coping with trauma.

Health Consequences and Awareness

The long-term health consequences of radiation exposure were another critical lesson. Survivors experienced a range of health issues, including increased incidences of cancer, chronic illnesses, and psychological disorders. The hibakusha's experiences underscore the need for ongoing health monitoring and care for those exposed to nuclear fallout. They have advocated for awareness regarding the dangers of radiation, the importance of scientific research on its effects, and the necessity of healthcare access for affected individuals.

Advocacy for Peace and Nuclear Disarmament
One of the most significant lessons from Hiroshima and Nagasaki is the urgency of advocating for nuclear disarmament and peace. Many survivors have become vocal activists, sharing their stories to raise awareness about the horrors of nuclear war and to prevent future occurrences. Their testimonies serve as powerful reminders of the human cost of nuclear weapons and the importance of diplomatic efforts to resolve conflicts without resorting to violence. The hibakusha's resolve to promote peace has inspired global movements focused on disarmament and non-proliferation, illustrating how personal experiences can lead to collective action.

Building Community Resilience
Survivors also highlight the importance of community resilience in the face of disaster. In the aftermath of the bombings, communities came together to support one another, sharing resources and providing emotional support. This sense of community played a vital role in recovery and rebuilding efforts. Hibakusha stress that fostering strong community ties is essential not only for coping with immediate crises but also for ensuring long-term recovery and resilience.

Conclusion
The lessons learned from the atomic bombings of Hiroshima and Nagasaki are invaluable in today's world, where nuclear threats persist. The experiences of the hibakusha remind us of the profound consequences of nuclear warfare and the importance of preparedness, mental health support, and advocacy for peace. By reflecting on their stories, we can better understand the complexities of survival in the face of catastrophic events and the fundamental need to strive for a world free from the threat of nuclear weapons.

The Cuban Missile Crisis: Avoiding Nuclear Catastrophe
The Cuban Missile Crisis of October 1962 remains one of the most precarious moments in the history of international relations, highlighting how close the world came to nuclear war. This 13-day confrontation between the United States and the Soviet Union arose from the discovery of Soviet nuclear missiles stationed in Cuba, just 90 miles off the coast of Florida. The crisis was a culmination of escalating tensions during the Cold War, marked by a series of geopolitical maneuvers that left both superpowers on edge.

The roots of the crisis can be traced back to earlier events, including the failed Bay of Pigs invasion in April 1961, which aimed to overthrow the Cuban government led by Fidel Castro. In response to this perceived threat, Castro sought support from the Soviet Union, culminating in the placement of nuclear missiles in Cuba. U.S. intelligence, through aerial reconnaissance, confirmed the presence of these missiles on October 14, 1962, leading to a series of tense deliberations among President John F. Kennedy and his advisors.

Faced with the imminent threat of nuclear missiles within striking distance of the U.S. mainland, Kennedy convened a series of meetings known as the Executive Committee of the National Security Council (ExComm). The dilemma was profound: a military invasion to remove the missiles could prompt a Soviet response, potentially sparking a full-scale nuclear war. Conversely, doing nothing could embolden Soviet aggression. After extensive discussions, Kennedy opted for a naval blockade, termed a "quarantine," to prevent further shipments of military equipment to Cuba. This decision was critical, as it provided a non-confrontational approach while demonstrating U.S. resolve.

During the blockade, tensions escalated. Both nations prepared for possible military engagement, and the world held its breath as the threat of nuclear war loomed. The crisis reached its peak on October 27, when a U.S. U-2 reconnaissance plane was shot down over Cuba, and it was feared that a retaliatory strike could be imminent. However, it was at this critical juncture that back-channel communications between the U.S. and the Soviet Union proved invaluable. Secret negotiations unfolded, revealing a path to de-escalation.

The resolution came when the United States agreed to withdraw its Jupiter missiles from Turkey, which were positioned threateningly close to the Soviet Union, in exchange for the removal of Soviet missiles from Cuba. This compromise, though not publicly acknowledged at the time, effectively diffused the situation and averted disaster.

The Cuban Missile Crisis underscored the importance of communication and diplomacy in international relations, particularly in times of heightened tension. The establishment of the Moscow-Washington hotline following the crisis aimed to facilitate direct communication between the leaders of the two superpowers, reducing the risk of misunderstanding in future conflicts.

Ultimately, the crisis served as a wake-up call regarding the dangers of nuclear proliferation and the necessity for arms control. It led to subsequent treaties aimed at curbing nuclear weapons development, including the Limited Test Ban Treaty of 1963. The lessons learned from the Cuban Missile Crisis resonate today, as ongoing geopolitical tensions and the threat of nuclear conflict continue to challenge global stability.

In conclusion, the Cuban Missile Crisis was a pivotal moment in Cold War history that highlighted the precarious balance of power and the thin line between peace and nuclear catastrophe. The actions taken by both U.S. and Soviet leaders not only averted a potential disaster but also set the stage for future diplomatic efforts aimed at preventing nuclear war. The legacy of this crisis reminds us of the vital importance of dialogue, negotiation, and preparedness in the face of existential threats.

Chernobyl and Fukushima: Lessons from Nuclear Disasters

The catastrophic nuclear accidents at Chernobyl in 1986 and Fukushima in 2011 provide critical insights into managing radiation exposure and survival in the aftermath of a nuclear disaster. Both events, while differing in nature and context, highlight the importance of preparedness, effective response strategies, and long-term recovery planning in the face of nuclear hazards.

Understanding the Accidents

Chernobyl, located in the then-Soviet Union, was the result of a flawed reactor design coupled with severe violations of operational protocols. The explosion at Reactor No. 4 released a massive amount of radioactive material into the atmosphere, leading to widespread contamination and the eventual evacuation of over 100,000 people. In contrast, the Fukushima Daiichi nuclear disaster, triggered by a massive earthquake and tsunami, resulted in reactor meltdowns and significant releases of radiation. Despite having robust safety systems, the scale of the natural disaster overwhelmed the facility's defenses.

Immediate Response and Evacuation

One of the most significant lessons from both disasters is the critical importance of timely and efficient evacuation. In Chernobyl, the initial response was hampered by a lack of information and transparency, delaying the evacuation of nearby residents. This resulted in many individuals receiving high doses of radiation before they could reach safety. Conversely, Fukushima's response was more structured, with authorities implementing evacuation orders based on real-time radiation monitoring. The importance of having clear communication channels and evacuation plans cannot be overstated, as they can drastically reduce exposure and save lives.

Managing Radiation Exposure

Both events underscore the necessity of understanding and managing radiation exposure. In the aftermath of Chernobyl, the phenomenon of "liquidators" emerged, comprised of emergency workers who were exposed to high radiation levels while responding to the crisis. Many suffered from acute radiation sickness and long-term health effects. Similarly, in Fukushima, workers faced the challenge of operating in contaminated environments, highlighting the need for adequate training and protective measures.

Survivors and responders must be educated about radiation's effects, including the symptoms of exposure and the importance of decontamination. Individuals should be equipped with personal dosimeters to monitor exposure levels, allowing them to make informed decisions about their safety.

Long-Term Health Monitoring and Psychological Impact
Long-term health monitoring is crucial for those exposed to radiation. Chernobyl survivors have shown increased rates of thyroid cancer and other health issues, necessitating ongoing medical support and research to understand the long-term impacts of radiation exposure. Similarly, the psychological effects of both disasters have been profound, with many survivors experiencing anxiety, depression, and post-traumatic stress disorder (PTSD). Mental health support must be included in disaster preparedness plans to help individuals cope with the trauma and uncertainties following a nuclear incident.

Community Resilience and Recovery
Chernobyl and Fukushima also serve as powerful examples of community resilience. In the wake of these disasters, affected communities have demonstrated remarkable strength in rebuilding their lives. The establishment of support networks, both locally and globally, plays a pivotal role in recovery. Community education programs focused on emergency preparedness and radiation safety can empower individuals to take proactive measures in the face of potential nuclear threats.

Conclusion
The lessons drawn from the Chernobyl and Fukushima disasters emphasize the importance of preparedness, timely response, and ongoing support for affected individuals. By learning from these events, societies can better equip themselves to manage the challenges posed by nuclear incidents, ensuring that both immediate and long-term needs are effectively addressed. Understanding the complexities of radiation exposure and the psychological impacts of such traumatic events is crucial for fostering resilience and promoting recovery in any future nuclear disaster scenario.

The Cold War Bunkers: Preparedness and Paranoia
The Cold War era, spanning from the late 1940s to the early 1990s, was marked by intense geopolitical rivalry, particularly between the United States and the Soviet Union. This period fostered a pervasive culture of fear and paranoia regarding nuclear warfare, profoundly influencing public consciousness and survival strategies. The threat of nuclear annihilation loomed over daily life, prompting governments and civilians alike to take drastic measures to prepare for a potential nuclear conflict.

Development of Bunkers

In response to the escalating tensions and the arms race, nations invested heavily in the construction of bunkers designed to protect against nuclear attacks. These bunkers varied widely in size and sophistication, from small private shelters built in backyards to large, government-constructed facilities capable of housing thousands. In the United States, projects such as the Greenbrier bunker, hidden beneath a luxury hotel in West Virginia, were built to protect government officials in the event of a nuclear strike. The Soviet Union, too, constructed vast underground complexes intended to shelter military personnel and civilians.

The architectural designs of these bunkers were heavily influenced by the knowledge of nuclear physics. Engineers had to consider factors such as blast waves, thermal radiation, and radioactive fallout. Consequently, bunkers were fortified with thick concrete walls and were often equipped with air filtration systems to mitigate the effects of nuclear fallout. The emphasis on creating self-sufficient environments was critical; many bunkers included supplies for food, water, and medical care, reflecting a belief that survival would require isolation from the outside world.

Civil Defense Initiatives

Beyond government initiatives, the Cold War prompted widespread civil defense programs aimed at educating the public on nuclear preparedness. Governments organized drills, disseminated literature, and promoted "duck and cover" campaigns that instructed civilians on how to react in the event of a nuclear explosion. Schools held regular drills where students practiced taking cover under desks, while families were encouraged to create emergency plans and stockpile supplies.

In the United States, the Federal Civil Defense Administration (FCDA) played a crucial role in these efforts, producing pamphlets and films to instill a sense of preparedness among citizens. Campaigns often emphasized the idea that individuals could survive a nuclear attack if they were properly equipped and educated. This fostered a societal belief in personal agency in the face of impending doom, albeit within the confines of a highly paranoid environment.

Cultural Impact

The paranoia of the Cold War era permeated popular culture, manifesting in films, literature, and art that depicted nuclear catastrophe and survival. Movies such as "Dr. Strangelove" and "The Day After" reflected societal anxieties about nuclear conflict and the absurdity of the arms race. These portrayals both entertained and instilled fear, reinforcing the notion that nuclear war was not just a distant possibility but an imminent threat.

Moreover, the psychological impact of constant fear of nuclear war led to a societal obsession with preparedness. Many families constructed backyard bunkers, stocked up on canned goods, and kept gas masks at the ready, embodying the belief that self-reliance was essential for survival. This culture of preparedness was both a response to real geopolitical tensions and a reflection of the psychological burden of living under the threat of nuclear annihilation.

Conclusion

The legacy of Cold War bunkers and the associated culture of preparedness and paranoia has had a lasting impact on contemporary survival strategies. While the immediate threat of nuclear war may have diminished since the end of the Cold War, the lessons learned during this tumultuous period remain relevant. The emphasis on preparedness, resilience, and community collaboration in the face of existential threats continues to inform how societies approach potential modern crises, reflecting a historical understanding that, in the end, survival often hinges not just on physical shelter but on collective awareness and action.

Modern Nuclear Threats: North Korea and Iran

The proliferation of nuclear weapons remains one of the most pressing global challenges of the 21st century. Among the nations currently posing significant nuclear threats, North Korea and Iran stand out due to their contentious geopolitical stances, nuclear ambitions, and the implications of their arsenals for international security. Understanding these threats and the global responses is crucial in navigating the complexities of modern nuclear politics.

North Korea: A Persistent Threat

North Korea's nuclear ambitions have escalated dramatically since its first nuclear test in 2006, positioning it as a critical threat not just to regional stability in East Asia but also to global security. The Kim regime has pursued nuclear weapons as a means of deterrence against perceived external threats, particularly from the United States and South Korea. This pursuit has led to a series of provocative missile tests and nuclear detonations, raising alarms internationally.

The North Korean government's insistence on maintaining its nuclear arsenal is rooted in its strategy of "byungjin," which aims to advance both economic and nuclear capabilities simultaneously. Despite international sanctions, North Korea has demonstrated resilience in its nuclear development, reportedly achieving advancements in missile technology and nuclear yield. The potential for these weapons to reach U.S. territory, coupled with the regime's unpredictable behavior, has compelled the international community to seek various diplomatic and military responses.

Iran: The Nuclear Enigma

Iran's nuclear program has similarly raised concerns, particularly regarding its potential to develop nuclear weapons capabilities. The country insists its program is for peaceful purposes; however, the opacity surrounding its nuclear activities has led to widespread suspicion. The 2015 Joint Comprehensive Plan of Action (JCPOA) was a significant diplomatic effort to limit Iran's nuclear capabilities in exchange for sanctions relief. Under this agreement, Iran agreed to restrict its enrichment activities and allow extensive inspections.

However, the U.S. withdrawal from the JCPOA in 2018, followed by the re-imposition of sanctions, has led Iran to gradually breach the agreement's limits, enriching uranium to levels closer to weapons-grade. This escalation has heightened fears of a nuclear arms race in the Middle East, particularly involving nations such as Saudi Arabia and Israel, which view a nuclear-capable Iran as an existential threat.

Global Responses and Challenges

The responses to the nuclear threats posed by North Korea and Iran have varied significantly, reflecting the complexities of international diplomacy. In the case of North Korea, the U.S. has employed a strategy of "maximum pressure," combining sanctions with diplomatic overtures, including high-profile summits between U.S. and North Korean leaders. However, these efforts have yielded mixed results, and the region remains on edge, with military options still debated among policymakers.

For Iran, the re-engagement in diplomacy represents a potential path forward, but the lack of trust and the geopolitical realities of the Middle East complicate negotiations. The international community, including the European Union and regional partners, has sought to mediate and restore some form of agreement, but the path to a sustainable resolution is fraught with challenges.

Conclusion

The nuclear threats from North Korea and Iran exemplify the multifaceted challenges of modern nuclear proliferation. They underscore the need for robust international cooperation, diplomatic engagement, and strategic deterrence to prevent escalation. As these countries continue to develop their nuclear capabilities, the global community must remain vigilant and proactive in its responses, balancing sanctions, diplomacy, and security measures to mitigate the risks of nuclear conflict. Understanding the intricacies of these threats is essential for fostering a safer and more stable world in the face of rising nuclear tensions.

Chapter 20

Conclusion

Reflecting on the Lessons Learned

In the face of an ever-evolving global landscape fraught with the threat of nuclear conflict, the lessons gleaned from history and preparation become essential for survival. "How to Survive a Nuclear War" serves as a comprehensive guide that not only addresses the mechanics of survival in the event of a nuclear catastrophe but also emphasizes the importance of understanding the broader implications of nuclear warfare. This reflection on the lessons learned highlights key takeaways crucial for individuals and communities in preparing for and responding to nuclear threats.

1. Understanding the Nature of the Threat:

The historical context of nuclear weapons development underscores the urgency of comprehending their destructive potential. The horrifying experiences of Hiroshima and Nagasaki remind us that the consequences of nuclear conflict are not merely theoretical; they are real and devastating. Acknowledging the history of nuclear warfare and its aftermath equips individuals with a sobering awareness of what is at stake, fostering a culture of preparedness rather than complacency.

2. The Importance of Community Preparedness:

Survival in a nuclear crisis is not solely an individual endeavor. The book emphasizes the significance of community networks—how collective preparedness can enhance resilience. By building communication systems, organizing local resources, and fostering relationships, communities can create a support system that extends beyond individual survival. This interconnectedness can facilitate effective resource management, emotional support, and the sharing of knowledge, all of which are vital during a crisis.

3. Mental and Emotional Resilience:

Psychological preparedness is highlighted as a critical component of surviving a nuclear event. The emotional toll of such an experience can be profound, leading to long-lasting trauma. The book offers strategies for coping with the psychological impacts of a nuclear crisis, stressing the necessity of mental health care and the importance of maintaining hope. Cultivating resilience through coping mechanisms, community support, and spiritual practices can help individuals navigate the challenges of post-nuclear life.

4. Practical Skills and Resource Management:

In the aftermath of a nuclear event, knowledge of practical skills becomes invaluable. The ability to purify water, grow food, and manage resources effectively can mean the difference between life and death. The book emphasizes the necessity of learning these skills before an emergency arises, enabling individuals to adapt to a new reality with confidence. It advocates for a proactive approach in acquiring knowledge and practicing survival techniques, ensuring preparedness for a variety of scenarios.

5. Ethical Considerations and Moral Readiness:

The discussion surrounding ethics in survival situations is a poignant reminder that the human experience does not cease in the face of catastrophe. The book encourages readers to consider the moral complexities of survival, emphasizing compassion and empathy even in dire circumstances. Preparing for ethical dilemmas fosters a mindset that values community and humanity, essential for rebuilding society after a nuclear disaster.

6. Continuous Vigilance and Adaptation:

Finally, one of the most crucial lessons learned is the importance of ongoing vigilance. The geopolitical landscape is dynamic, and the threat of nuclear conflict may evolve. Staying informed about global affairs, understanding governmental responses, and remaining adaptable to new information are vital for effective preparation. This proactive stance not only enhances individual and community resilience but also contributes to a larger dialogue about nuclear disarmament and global peace.

In conclusion, the reflections on the lessons learned from "How to Survive a Nuclear War" serve as a clarion call for awareness, preparedness, and resilience. By internalizing these teachings, individuals and communities can cultivate a robust foundation to navigate the complexities of potential nuclear threats while fostering hope for a more peaceful future. The journey towards survival is not simply about enduring a catastrophe; it is also about learning, adapting, and ultimately thriving in the face of adversity.

The Importance of Preparedness and Vigilance

In an increasingly complex global landscape, the specter of nuclear conflict remains a pressing concern. The reality that nations possess vast arsenals of nuclear weapons underscores the necessity for individuals and communities to maintain a state of preparedness and vigilance. The importance of ongoing preparation can be broken down into several key areas: risk mitigation, mental resilience, effective response, and community cohesion.

Risk Mitigation

Preparedness is fundamentally about risk management. By understanding the potential threats and preparing for them, individuals can significantly reduce their vulnerability to catastrophic events. This involves not only acquiring knowledge about nuclear weapons and their effects but also developing comprehensive emergency plans tailored to specific risks faced by one's community. Whether it's creating a family emergency kit stocked with essentials or establishing clear communication plans, thoughtful risk mitigation strategies empower individuals to respond effectively in the face of uncertainty.

Mental Resilience

The psychological impact of a nuclear threat can be overwhelming. Preparedness fosters mental resilience, equipping individuals with the tools to cope with anxiety and fear. Awareness of potential scenarios and practicing emergency responses can alleviate feelings of helplessness. Engaging in preparedness activities—such as community drills or family discussions about safety—can cultivate a sense of agency and control. This proactive approach helps alleviate panic and confusion during an actual crisis, allowing individuals to make rational decisions instead of succumbing to fear.

Effective Response

In the event of a nuclear incident, the first hours are critical. Preparedness can mean the difference between life and death. Knowing how to recognize warning signs, where to find immediate shelter, and how to protect oneself from radiation can save lives. Training and education about the appropriate actions to take during a nuclear event enable individuals and families to act swiftly and efficiently. This preparedness extends to understanding the nuances of communication during a crisis and the importance of staying informed through reliable channels.

Community Cohesion

No individual is an island, and the strength of a community can significantly enhance overall preparedness. Fostering a culture of preparedness within neighborhoods and local organizations creates a network of support that can be invaluable during emergencies. Community drills, workshops, and planning sessions encourage collective awareness and resource sharing. A well-prepared community can coordinate aid, share information, and provide emotional support, thus enhancing the resilience of its members. Moreover, communal preparedness initiatives can help bridge social divides, fostering collaboration and strengthening community bonds in the face of adversity.

Maintaining Awareness

Preparedness is not a one-time event but a continuous process. The global political landscape is dynamic, and threats can evolve rapidly. Keeping abreast of current events, understanding international relations, and actively engaging in discussions about nuclear policy are vital for maintaining an informed perspective. This ongoing awareness encourages individuals to advocate for policies that promote disarmament and conflict resolution, thereby contributing to a safer world.

Conclusion

In conclusion, the importance of preparedness and vigilance cannot be overstated in a world where the threat of nuclear conflict looms. By investing time and effort into understanding risks, developing effective responses, and fostering community cohesion, individuals not only enhance their own survival prospects but also contribute to the broader goal of societal resilience. Ultimately, a well-prepared populace is a cornerstone of security, capable of navigating the complexities of a post-nuclear world with greater confidence and unity. In a landscape fraught with uncertainty, ongoing preparation and awareness are not merely advisable; they are essential.

Rebuilding a Better World: Hope and Optimism

In the aftermath of a nuclear event, the immediate landscape is often one of chaos, fear, and uncertainty. However, amidst the rubble and despair, the seeds of hope and optimism can be sown to cultivate a future that not only rebuilds what was lost but also improves upon the past. This section explores the principles and strategies for fostering a resilient and cohesive society in the wake of destruction.

Embracing Community Resilience

The foundation for rebuilding a better world lies in the strength and unity of communities. After a nuclear event, individuals often find themselves isolated and overwhelmed. It is critical to foster a sense of community resilience, wherein individuals come together to support one another. This can be achieved through local gatherings, resource-sharing initiatives, and collaborative problem-solving. By creating strong networks of mutual aid, communities can pool their resources, skills, and knowledge, making them more adaptable in the face of adversity.

Learning from the Past

Drawing lessons from history is paramount in the rebuilding process. Survivors of past nuclear events, such as Hiroshima and Nagasaki, provide invaluable insights into the psychological and social strategies that aided their recovery. Understanding how these communities navigated the complexities of loss, trauma, and rebuilding can inform current efforts. It is essential to document and share these stories, as they serve as both cautionary tales and sources of inspiration. The experiences of those who endured significant hardships can illuminate pathways toward healing and reconstruction.

Fostering Innovation and Sustainability

Rebuilding after a nuclear event presents an opportunity to reimagine societal structures and prioritize sustainable practices. The devastation can serve as a catalyst for innovation, prompting societies to explore new technologies and methods that are not only efficient but also environmentally responsible. Emphasizing renewable energy, sustainable agriculture, and waste reduction can help create a resilient infrastructure that mitigates the risk of future crises. By investing in green technologies and practices, communities can rebuild in a way that protects the planet and fosters long-term sustainability.

Encouraging Inclusive Governance

A vital aspect of rebuilding a better world is the establishment of inclusive governance. In the aftermath of a nuclear event, there may be a temptation for authoritarian structures to emerge in response to chaos. However, inclusivity and participation are essential for effective governance. Engaging diverse voices in decision-making processes ensures that the needs and concerns of all community members are addressed. Transparent governance that prioritizes accountability and justice can foster trust and cooperation among citizens, paving the way for a more equitable society.

Cultivating Hope Through Education

Education plays a crucial role in fostering a culture of hope and optimism. In the wake of destruction, educational initiatives should focus not only on knowledge transfer but also on emotional and psychological support. Teaching resilience, problem-solving, and critical thinking can empower individuals to navigate the complexities of a post-nuclear world. Furthermore, integrating lessons on peace, cooperation, and conflict resolution into curricula can promote a culture of understanding, reducing the likelihood of future conflicts.

Building a Culture of Compassion

Ultimately, rebuilding a better world hinges on cultivating a culture of compassion and empathy. In times of crisis, the human spirit often shines brightest through acts of kindness and solidarity. Encouraging individuals to engage in volunteerism, mentorship, and community service can foster connections and a sense of belonging. By prioritizing compassion in every aspect of rebuilding—be it in governance, education, or community initiatives—societies can create an environment that nurtures healing, understanding, and hope.

In conclusion, while the aftermath of a nuclear event may initially seem insurmountable, it presents a unique opportunity to rebuild a better world. By embracing community resilience, learning from the past, fostering innovation, encouraging inclusive governance, cultivating hope through education, and building a culture of compassion, societies can emerge from the ashes of destruction with renewed strength and purpose. The journey toward rebuilding is not merely about physical reconstruction but about creating a more just, equitable, and hopeful future for all.

The Future of Nuclear Weapons: Challenges and Opportunities

The landscape of nuclear weapons is undergoing profound transformations as the world grapples with evolving geopolitical tensions, technological advancements, and the pressing need for disarmament. The future of nuclear weapons will be shaped by a complex interplay of challenges and opportunities that policymakers, scientists, and civil society must navigate to prevent catastrophic outcomes.

Challenges Ahead

One of the most significant challenges is the proliferation of nuclear capabilities. As more nations pursue nuclear weapons, the risk of nuclear conflict increases. Countries like North Korea have demonstrated that nuclear aspirations can be pursued even in the face of international sanctions and diplomatic pressure. This "nuclear proliferation" is fueled by regional tensions, national security concerns, and the desire for increased geopolitical influence. The challenge lies in creating effective frameworks to prevent further nuclear development while addressing the underlying political issues that drive nations to seek these capabilities.

Another pressing challenge is the modernization of existing nuclear arsenals. Many nuclear-armed states are investing heavily in upgrading their weapons systems, which includes developing new delivery methods, enhancing warhead reliability, and integrating advanced technologies like artificial intelligence. This modernization race threatens to undermine existing arms control treaties and could lead to a new arms race reminiscent of the Cold War era. The potential for miscalculation during crises, where states may feel pressured to use or threaten the use of nuclear weapons, remains a grave concern.

Opportunities for Change

Despite these challenges, there are numerous opportunities on the horizon that can reshape the future of nuclear weapons. One such opportunity lies in the revitalization of international arms control agreements. Treaties like the Treaty on the Non-Proliferation of Nuclear Weapons (NPT) and new bilateral agreements, such as those between the United States and Russia, provide platforms for dialogue and cooperation. Renewed commitment to these frameworks can lead to significant reductions in nuclear stockpiles and foster a culture of trust among nations.

Moreover, advancements in technology can play a dual role. While technologies such as cyber capabilities and missile defense systems can exacerbate tensions, they also offer potential pathways to enhance security. For instance, improving early warning systems and developing robust communication channels can help mitigate misunderstandings during crises, reducing the likelihood of accidental nuclear war. Additionally, international collaboration on nuclear nonproliferation technologies can lead to the sharing of best practices, enhancing global security.

The Role of Civil Society and Advocacy

The growing influence of civil society and grassroots movements advocating for nuclear disarmament presents another opportunity. Public awareness campaigns and advocacy efforts can pressure governments to take action on disarmament initiatives, create momentum for policy changes, and foster a culture that values peace over militarization. Initiatives like the Treaty on the Prohibition of Nuclear Weapons (TPNW) exemplify how civil society can influence international norms regarding nuclear weapons, pushing for a future where these weapons are viewed as an unacceptable threat to humanity.

Final Thoughts

The future of nuclear weapons is fraught with challenges that require urgent attention and innovative solutions. However, opportunities exist to reshape the global nuclear landscape through renewed diplomatic efforts, technological advancements, and the active involvement of civil society. By prioritizing disarmament, enhancing international cooperation, and preparing for the ethical implications of advanced technologies, the global community can work towards a safer, more stable world free from the threat of nuclear annihilation. In this complex environment, the focus must remain on prevention, resilience, and the shared commitment to a future where nuclear weapons are no longer a tool of national security, but a relic of a bygone era.

Final Thoughts: Surviving and Thriving

As we conclude this exploration of nuclear survival, it is essential to reflect on the journey we've undertaken together. The threat of nuclear war, while daunting, is not insurmountable. By fostering a culture of awareness, preparedness, and community support, we can equip ourselves to face such challenges with resilience and determination. The path forward is not merely about surviving a catastrophe; it is about thriving in its aftermath and rebuilding a world that reflects our shared values of compassion and cooperation.

Continued Learning

Knowledge is our greatest ally in times of crisis. The landscape of global politics, technological advancements, and environmental conditions is constantly evolving. Therefore, it is vital to stay informed about current events, nuclear policies, and the scientific principles underlying nuclear weapons and their effects. Engage with credible sources of information, attend workshops, and participate in community preparedness drills. Learning from history—both the triumphs and tragedies—can provide invaluable insights into how we can better prepare for the future. The lessons learned from Hiroshima and Nagasaki, the Cuban Missile Crisis, and nuclear accidents remind us of the fragility of peace and the importance of vigilant diplomacy.

Preparation as a Community

Survival in the face of adversity is rarely an individual endeavor. Building strong, interconnected communities is essential for resilience. Encourage your family, friends, and neighbors to develop their own preparedness plans and engage in collective training exercises. Create local emergency response groups that can share resources, skills, and knowledge. A community that understands the importance of preparedness can support its members during a crisis, ensuring that no one faces the challenges of a nuclear event alone. This sense of solidarity can be a beacon of hope, fostering an environment where people feel empowered and cared for, even in the darkest times.

Emotional and Psychological Resilience

Coping with the psychological impacts of a nuclear threat is as crucial as physical survival. Encourage open discussions about fears, anxieties, and uncertainties surrounding nuclear warfare. Establish support networks that prioritize mental health, allowing individuals to share their experiences and feelings in a safe environment. By nurturing emotional resilience through mindfulness practices, community support, and constructive communication, we can better prepare ourselves and our loved ones for the psychological toll of a nuclear crisis.

Commitment to Ethical Principles

In the wake of a disaster, ethical dilemmas may arise that test our values and humanity. It is essential to cultivate a mindset that emphasizes empathy, compassion, and cooperation. Engage in dialogues about moral challenges we may face in a post-nuclear society, and work towards solutions that prioritize the well-being of all. By committing to ethical principles, we not only enhance our chances of survival but also lay the groundwork for a more just and equitable society.

A Shared Vision for the Future

Finally, as we look to the future, let us envision a world that actively seeks to prevent nuclear conflict. Advocate for disarmament, support diplomatic solutions to international disputes, and promote education on the consequences of nuclear warfare. Each of us has a role to play in fostering peace and understanding among nations. By coming together, we can create a global culture that prioritizes dialogue over aggression and cooperation over division.

In conclusion, the journey of surviving and thriving in a post-nuclear world is not a solitary one. It requires a commitment to continuous learning, community engagement, emotional resilience, and ethical considerations. Together, we can forge a path that not only prepares us for potential crises but also nurtures a future defined by hope, compassion, and a shared commitment to rebuilding a better world.

Made in the USA
Middletown, DE
02 January 2025

68695100R00106